Caring for someone who has had a stroke

Philip Coyne with Penny Mares

AGE *Concern*

BOOKS

© 1995 Philip Coyne and Penny Mares
Published by Age Concern England
1268 London Road
London SW16 4ER

First published 1995 in Age Concern Books' *Caring in a Crisis* series
This edition published 1998
Reprinted 1999

Editor Caroline Hartnell
Production Vinnette Marshall
Designed and typeset by GreenGate Publishing Services, Tonbridge, Kent
Printed in Great Britain by Bell & Bain Ltd, Glasgow

A catalogue record for this book is available from the British Library.

ISBN 0-86242-264-7

Bulk orders

Age Concern England is pleased to offer customised editions of all its titles to UK
companies, institutions or other organisations wishing to make a bulk purchase.
For further information, please contact the Publishing Department at the address
above. Tel: 0181-679 8000. Fax: 0181-679 6069. E-mail: addisom@ace.org.uk

Contents

About the authors

Philip Coyne is an experienced researcher, writer and editor working primarily in the field of health and social concerns. His writing involves the presentation of technical subjects in a way that is accessible to a wide readership. He is an experienced writer and editor of open learning materials.

Recent work includes: editing *Our City, Our Health* for Sheffield Health Authority and Sheffield City Council; researching for and writing the health and safety unit for the Open College's New Supervisor series; researching for and writing *The Last Cigarette* booklet for Yorkshire Television; writing *First Aid in Coal Mines*, an open learning module for British Coal; editing *Children First* materials for the Child Care and Education NVQ; and writing *Roadcraft*, the police driver's handbook for the Association of Chief Police Officers and HMSO.

Philip's father died of a stroke, and he himself was diagnosed with hypertension at the age of 29. He has two children and lives in Yorkshire.

Penny Mares is an established writer on health issues. She has written a range of information and training materials for people caring at home. She is author of *You and Caring* published by the King's Fund and co-author of *Who Cares Now*, the book which accompanies the BBC TV series of the same name on caring for an older person. Penny also wrote *Caring for someone who is dying*, another book in this series 'Carers Handbook'.

Acknowledgements

We thank the following for their helpful comments and suggestions about this book. The final content of the book is, of course, the authors' responsibility.

John and Brenda Comben

Jack and Betty Whittard

Dr John and Mary Bavington

The members of Shipley Stroke Club

Elizabeth Baker, Yorkshire and Humberside Information Officer, The Stroke Association

Liz Ward, Principal Occupational Therapist, Leeds Social Services

Lesley Wood, Carers Development Officer, Leeds Social Services

Professor G Mulley, Consultant Physician, St James University Hospital, Leeds

Dr A House, Consultant in Liaison Psychiatry, Leeds General Infirmary

Dr J Bamford, Consultant Neurologist and Cerebrovascular Physician, St James University Hospital, Leeds

The Stroke Association

Introduction

Every year about 100,000 people in Britain will have a stroke; of these, about 70 per cent will survive the first few days and start to rebuild their lives. In rebuilding their lives they will rely heavily on the support of others – mainly their close relatives or friends. It is for these carers, often older people themselves, that this book has been written. Although written with carers in mind,the central concern of the book is people who have had a stroke. Hopefully, they too will find the book informative, useful and interesting.

What do we know about stroke? We know that it affects men slightly more than women; that, although it can occur at any age, about 80 per cent of the people affected are over 65; that most people who have a stroke will survive it; that 20 per cent of these people will be living alone; and that after one year about two-thirds of survivors will have regained independence in daily activities.

We also know that the effects of stroke may be devastating, the more so because it comes out of the blue; that its disruption affects not only the person involved but also their families; and that recovery from stroke may take time and may significantly change the lives of everyone involved. We know that recovery can be a slow and demanding process, but that rapid and complete recoveries are possible and that the achievements of many survivors and their carers are an inspiration to us all.

At any one time there are about 350,000 people in Britain who are rebuilding their lives after stroke. Typically they and their carers have three major hurdles to overcome. The first is the onset of stroke and its immediate aftermath, the second is discharge from hospital and adjustment to life at home, and the third is the end of hospital support and the feelings of isolation and abandonment that this often produces.

This book is designed to help you at each of these potential crisis points. It gives you the information you need at each stage to understand what is going on and what you can do about it, but most importantly it lets you know that you are not alone. There are professional groups and voluntary organisations that can give you support at every stage but, regrettably, you may not get this support unless you ask for it.

The book has nine chapters, a glossary and a list of useful addresses. If an organisation is mentioned in the text without an address, look for it in the Useful Addresses section at the back of the book. Recommendations on further reading are given at the end of each chapter.

Chapter 1 gives a general introduction to stroke, its causes and what you can do to reduce the risk of having one. Chapter 2 gives advice on what to do when your relative has a stroke, and looks at the important questions of where your relative should be cared for immediately after the stroke – at home or in hospital. Chapter 3 looks at the brain and why strokes have the effects that they do; it goes on to look at the common physical, psychological, emotional and social effects of stroke. Chapter 4 looks at the pattern and likelihood of recovery from stroke. It has advice on what you can do to help recovery and rehabilitation, and explains which professionals are likely to be involved in providing health and social care.

Chapter 5 helps you to plan for your relative's discharge from hospital, explains the role of community care in providing support and advises on arranging adequate support for your relative's return home. Chapter 6 looks at the practical and emotional issues that you need to consider when deciding on care for your relative. It looks at your needs as a carer, and the importance of adequate respite care. Chapter 7 gives advice on the everyday problems that arise when caring for your relative at home. It has advice on common psychological and emotional problems, including the sometimes difficult area of sex. It advises on where to get practical help with caring, how to use community care, how to deal with social service departments and where to get advice on the benefits that you and your relative may be entitled to.

Chapter 8 gives advice on how you can help with your relative's rehabilitation, the role of the professionals in rehabilitation and how to cope with the difficult time when professional help ends. Chapter 9 is about looking forward to the future. It gives advice on developing a healthy, positive life-style and reminds you as a carer of the importance of caring for yourself.

Because this book is written primarily for carers and because overwhelmingly carers are relatives, we generally refer in this book to the person who has had a stroke as *your relative*. We hope that other readers, especially those who have suffered a stroke, will not take offence because none is intended. We have also adopted the use of 'she' throughout some chapters and 'he' throughout others. There is no medical significance in this; it is merely a way of avoiding the rather clumsy 'he or she'.

1 What is stroke?

Most people know something about the effects of stroke – that it slurs speech or restricts the use of limbs – but they are not sure how this happens. If you are caring for someone whom you know is at risk of having a stroke, or who has had one, you need information. Understanding what a stroke is can help you to reduce the risks in future. It can help you make sense of the kinds of disabilities that result, and the problems that your relative may face in overcoming them. It can also help you work out how best to encourage and support your relative during recovery and rehabilitation.

This chapter explains what happens during a stroke, and how it is caused. It explains what factors affect the risk of stroke, and ways of reducing the risks. Finally, it explains the stages of recovering from a stroke.

Elizabeth

'He fell flat on the floor and couldn't get up, and that's where I found him.'

'I heard a thump and then Tom calling for me. I found him lying by the bed, looking frightened.

'A few weeks before, Tom's right arm and leg had gone numb for about 15 minutes and he'd been a bit confused. I was worried and said he should

1

see the doctor. He'd meant to go but he didn't. Then that Sunday morning his right arm went funny again, and as he got out of bed his leg collapsed. He fell flat on the floor and couldn't get up, and that's where I found him. The doctor said he'd had a stroke. His right arm and leg were paralysed and he couldn't speak properly, but now he's much better.'

What happens during a stroke?

A stroke happens when arteries supplying blood to the brain either get blocked (thrombosis) or burst (causing bleeding, or haemorrhage). Blockage cuts off the blood supply to part of the brain, and, without the oxygen and nutrients carried by the blood, brain cells stop working. If brain cells lose their blood supply for more than four to eight minutes, they die and cease working permanently. If a stroke is caused by a burst blood vessel, blood goes into the brain tissue, causing damage to brain cells.

Brain cells are like offices in the headquarters of a large organisation. Each office has its own specialised task. Offices are grouped into sections to cover larger task areas. If, suddenly, a number of offices or sections are shut down, their tasks no longer get done. The bigger the area that is shut down, the greater the disruption. In the long run other offices may take over some of the tasks but there will be a limit to what they can do.

The brain is organised into specialised areas of cells. Each has its own jobs to do. When an area of the brain dies because the blood supply has been interrupted, the jobs it performs are no longer done. In the long term, other areas of the brain may take over some of these jobs, but it can be a slow and uncertain process.

Because our brains control what we think, what we do and the functioning of our bodies, the death of cells in any area of our brains can have serious effects. Depending on where the damage is, emotions, understanding, memory, speech, sight, reading and writing, balance, walking, arm movement, muscle control, continence and other bodily functions can be affected, though usually not all together.

What causes stroke?

Stroke is caused by an interruption in the supply of blood to the brain. Four arteries feed the brain with blood: one each side of the neck (the left and right internal carotid arteries), and one up each side of the spine (the left and right vertebral arteries). These arteries link together at the base of the brain to form a joint supply for the brain. The two vertebral arteries join to form the basilar artery. This then joins the two internal carotid arteries to form a circle of arteries (the circle of Willis). Smaller arteries lead off from the circle of Willis and divide into smaller vessels called arterioles. These lead into capillaries which form a network of vessels supplying the brain with blood.

Because the four arteries supplying the brain are linked in this central circle of arteries, the effects of a blockage in one artery are minimised. If one of the internal carotid or vertebral arteries gets blocked, the other three arteries can sometimes supply enough blood to the circle of Willis to make good the loss. As age and disease progressively reduce the ability of the arteries to supply blood, it becomes more difficult for the unblocked arteries to make up any loss.

A stroke is caused by either a blockage of or bleeding from the arteries supplying the brain. A blockage or bleeding can occur anywhere in these arteries or in the very fine network of vessels that they eventually become. The bigger the vessel that is blocked or bursts, the more serious the effects.

Blockages

A **thrombosis** is a blockage caused by a solid clot of blood growing on the wall of an artery. The clot itself is called a **thrombus** and grows where the wall of the artery is damaged by disease.

An **embolism** is a clot of blood or other material that has formed somewhere else, broken away and moved through the arteries until it has come to a point that is too narrow for it to continue; at this

3

Arteries supplying blood to the brain

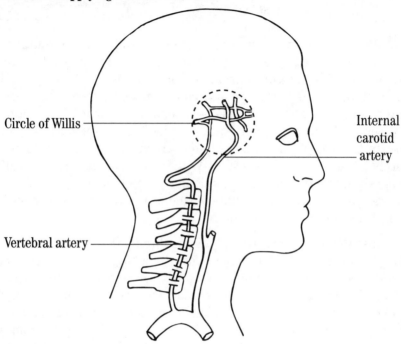

Circle of Willis

Internal
carotid
artery

Vertebral artery

The circle of Willis

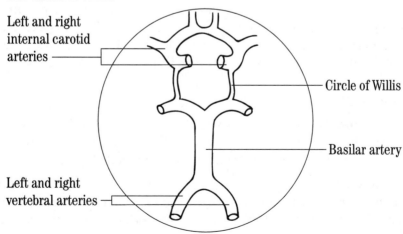

Left and right
internal carotid
arteries

Left and right
vertebral arteries

Circle of Willis

Basilar artery

point it jams and blocks the flow of blood through the artery. These clots usually form in the heart or in an artery in the neck and move up towards the brain. They are usually caused by heart or arterial disease.

Atherosclerosis (pronounced *ath-er-o-skler-o-sis*) is a hardening of the arteries combined with deposits of fat, cholesterol and other substances on their inner linings. It is a common cause of embolism and thrombosis. The disease narrows and damages the artery walls, which in turn encourages the growth of blood clots. As an artery narrows it restricts the flow of blood, and if a clot (thrombus) forms it can grow large enough to completely block the artery. Sometimes one of these clots breaks away from the inner lining of the artery and moves along it to cause an embolism elsewhere.

Atherosclerosis can affect all the arteries. When a blockage occurs in one artery supplying the brain, it is likely that the other arteries are also narrowed and unable to make up the shortfall in blood supply. Atherosclerosis can affect the arteries supplying the heart, causing heart disease. When the heart is damaged by disease, clots can form in it and float off to cause an embolism elsewhere. Other diseases of the heart such as **atrial fibrillation** (irregular heartbeat) can also cause clots which may break away to cause an embolism.

Bleeding into the brain (cerebral haemorrhage)

About 15 per cent of strokes in the UK are the result of bleeding into the brain (**cerebral haemorrhage**). These strokes can be severe because the part of the brain usually affected is the part that controls movement. The main cause is long-term high blood pressure (**hypertension**), or the formation of a small berry-like weak point (**berry aneurysm**) on the artery wall which enlarges and then bursts.

High blood pressure puts the arteries under stress and encourages the laying down of fat and other substances on the artery wall. Over time the arteries lose flexibility, which makes them more likely to burst. The resulting bleeding into the brain usually damages brain cells. High blood pressure can also contribute to the formation of aneurysms – where pressure forces a weak part of the artery wall to 'bubble out'. Eventually this weak area may burst, a bit like a blow-out on a car tyre. Aneurysms generally affect people over 50. Occasionally, young people are affected because they were born with a tendency to weakness in part of an artery wall.

Underlying causes of stroke

There are a number of things that increase the risk of a stroke:

- arterial disease
- diabetes
- excess blood cholesterol
- excess weight
- excessive alcohol
- excessive salt intake
- heart disease
- high blood pressure
- kidney disease
- lack of exercise
- old age
- smoking

The most important is high blood pressure. As you can see, some conditions are the result of unhealthy habits or life-style; others are long-term diseases not related to life-style. The effect of all of them is to damage the artery wall or to cause clotting, or both. Many of these conditions can be treated by drugs (eg high blood pressure, which responds well to treatment) or a by a change in life-style. None of them *inevitably* leads to a stroke, but they provide a warning of a greater than average risk. The more conditions that a person has, the greater the risk of a stroke. So, for example, smoking predisposes to stroke, but smoking combined with untreated high blood pressure puts you at greater risk. Diagnosis and treatment of these conditions can help prevent first or subsequent strokes.

Although stroke can occur at any age, 80 per cent of people who have a stroke are over 65. The older you get, the greater the risk, probably because hardening of the arteries increases and you are also more likely to have one of the conditions listed above. But even with age, a stroke is a risk, not a certainty. At 85 and over, only about four people out of every hundred are likely to have a stroke each year. For someone aged between 45 and 54, the risk is about one in a thousand.

Things that don't cause stroke

'I made myself miserable by taking things too far. I would go to a pub and I wouldn't have anything – I wouldn't have any beer because of the alcohol, I wouldn't have a single crisp because of the salt and fat. I wouldn't have a soft drink because of the sugar. I was bored and fed up and made everyone else feel the same. Then I went on a stroke club trip and I saw people with worse strokes than me enjoying themselves and having a drink. I said "you can't do that" and they said "why not?" I realised I spent all my time thinking about the next stroke. I'd convinced myself that unless I denied myself everything I was bound to have another one. I got more and more depressed until I saw the community psychiatric nurse. She helped me see things in perspective. I now enjoy life a lot more, and well I'm still here aren't I?'

Things like sudden physical exertion, overwork, stress, anger or an argument do *not* cause strokes although many people believe they do. After a tragic event like a stroke, it is a natural reaction to ask 'why me?' and to wonder if it was caused by anything you did. Looking for something to blame is a way of regaining control over the disruption of our lives, but it can also be a source of unnecessary guilt and unhappiness. We might say to ourselves things like 'If only I hadn't let Trevor paper the ceiling, he wouldn't have had a stroke.' But it is the underlying medical conditions that have built up over years that cause stroke, not a bout of temper or the physical effort of decorating.

There is some evidence that certain personality types are more likely than others to have a stroke. People with aggressive, competitive personalities do seem to suffer from increased risk of arterial disease and therefore stroke. But this is a long-term condition; occasional irritation at someone trying to push into a queue does not put you at greater risk. Occasionally a stroke occurs after a major emotional upset but this is probably because the upset triggers an event that would have happened anyway.

If you are caring for someone who has had a stroke, what are your own ideas about why it happened?

- Note them down on a piece of paper, especially the half-beliefs that you catch yourself musing on.
- Look at them and try to decide which are genuine reasons and which are not.
- If you cannot make up your mind, discuss them with someone else – perhaps your doctor, a relative or someone at the stroke club. These beliefs can be a source of unnecessary guilt, sapping your energies and undermining hope. They can also place unnecessary restrictions on your own or your relative's life, preventing you from doing things you would otherwise enjoy.

Warning signs of stroke

Most of the conditions listed on page 6 directly increase the risk of stroke. Excessive weight does not in itself increase the risk of stroke, but is often a sign that an individual has one of the medical conditions or life-style problems that do.

Transient ischaemic attack

One warning sign is a Transient Ischaemic Attack (TIA). Ischaemic (pronounced *is-key-mik*) means reduced blood supply. A TIA is like a small stroke. It comes on suddenly and lasts for less than 24 hours, usually between 5 and 30 minutes. What happens is that a clot of blood temporarily blocks the blood supply to part of the brain or eye. The blockage either is not big enough or does not last long enough to kill the cells, so they recover when the blood supply is restored. While the blood supply to the cells is reduced they stop working normally, and this gives rise to the symptoms of a TIA.

How to recognise a TIA

The symptoms are similar to a stroke, but wear off quickly. They can occur separately or in combination:

- blindness or blind spots in one eye or both
- difficulty in talking
- double vision and other distortions of sight
- left-sided blindness or right-sided blindness in both eyes
- numbness, weakness or tingling of an arm, leg, hand or foot
- numbness, weakness or tingling of one side of the face or body
- dizziness (vertigo)

These symptoms may have other causes that have nothing to do with stroke. In particular, blackouts, fainting and loss of consciousness are generally *not* symptoms of TIA.

Although the symptoms of TIA do not last long, someone who experiences them should see a doctor. It is important to get a proper diagnosis. There are several diseases with symptoms similar to those of TIA but which have different treatments. A TIA may be a warning of the risk of a more serious stroke or a heart attack. One in three people who have had a TIA will have a full stroke within three years. Doing something about the underlying conditions *does* help to reduce these risks and may prevent a more serious stroke.

What can be done to reduce the risk of stroke?

TIAs have may causes, including high blood pressure and the narrowing and temporary blockage of blood vessels. These problems need to be tackled to prevent another stroke. Some possible treatments and preventive measures are explained below. You and your relative may find these helpful if you want to ask questions or discuss

9

treatment with your doctor. If you feel that one of the options may have been overlooked, ask your doctor for more information.

High blood pressure (hypertension)

High blood pressure increases your susceptibility to stroke and other diseases (heart disease, coronary thrombosis and kidney problems). The higher your blood pressure, the more likely you are to have a stroke in the next five years, but high blood pressure is also the most treatable of the causes of stroke. If blood pressure is lowered, the risk of stroke is reduced. Drugs are the most effective way of lowering blood pressure, but changes in diet and an increase in exercise also help.

Blood pressure increases with age, but high blood pressure is generally defined as higher than 140 over 90. The top (**systolic**) reading gives the pressure when the heart beats; the bottom (**diastolic**) reading gives the pressure when the heart relaxes.

Someone who thinks he might be at risk from stroke should get his blood pressure checked by his GP. The doctor may also do other tests such as a blood test, urine test, electrocardiogram (ECG, a record of electrical impulses from the heart which tells doctors how well it is working) to identify the cause of the high blood pressure. If the doctor prescribes tablets to reduce the pressure, they should be taken regularly or the blood pressure will rise again.

Some blood pressure tablets can cause unpleasant side effects. If this happens, go back to the doctor and explain the problems, as it is vital to reduce blood pressure and keep it reduced. The effects of different medicines vary from person to person, so finding the right match between patient and medicine is rather a question of trial and error. A doctor will try different tablets until one is found that reduces blood pressure with least side effects.

Smoking

Smoking contributes to atherosclerosis by increasing the heart rate and raising the blood pressure. It increases the stickiness of certain blood cells, making them more likely to clot. It also produces carbon monoxide which reduces the blood's ability to carry oxygen. Someone who smokes 20 cigarettes a day is three times more likely to have a stroke than a non-smoker. Smoking combined with high blood pressure is particularly risky. (The only reason more smokers don't have strokes is that they die of heart disease or lung cancer first.)

The only way to give up smoking is to decide to stop. This isn't easy. It may take several attempts. Most people manage to stop without the help of things such as nicotine tablets or hypnotism, but encouragement and support do make a big difference. Some GPs and health centres run 'quit smoking' groups. Quit is an organisation that provides information and advice on how to stop (see Useful Addresses).

Eating too much salt

A high salt intake increases blood pressure. In some people, reducing the amount of salt eaten lowers blood pressure quite quickly. Don't add extra salt to food in cooking or at the table, and avoid highly salted foods such as crisps. Sometimes a salt low in sodium (eg Lo-salt) is recommended as an alternative but some research indicates that this makes no difference.

Eating too much fat

Too much animal fat increases the risk of arterial disease, especially in someone who has high blood cholesterol. (This can be checked by a simple blood test.) To reduce blood cholesterol, cut down the amount of total fat in the diet and replace saturated fats (animal fats such as milk, cheese, butter, lard and dripping) with polyunsaturated fats (polyunsaturated margarines, olive oil, corn oil or sunflower seed oil). Cut all visible fat off meat, use skimmed or semi-skimmed milk instead of full cream milk and cottage cheese instead of other cheeses. The aim is to make a significant change in the amount and type of fat in the normal diet. If this is done, eating the *occasional* cream cake or lamb chop does no harm.

Drinking too much alcohol

Drinking alcohol raises blood pressure. Moderate drinking – less than three units (or 1.5 pints of beer) for men or two for women a day – probably does no harm and possibly some good. Excessive drinking is harmful. There is some evidence that 'binge' drinking causes stroke directly through raised blood pressure.

The contraceptive pill

For most young women the medical benefits of taking the pill far outweigh the risks. But for women who themselves or whose close family members suffer from unusual hardening or narrowing of the arteries, or who suffer from severe migraines, there is a slight risk of stroke and it is probably safer to use some other form of contraceptive.

Reducing the risk of clotting

Drugs that thin the blood – aspirin and warfarin and other anticoagulants – help reduce the risk of a stroke from blood clots. There is evidence that people who have already had a stroke or a heart attack can reduce the risk of having a stroke by 25 per cent, by taking 75mg of aspirin (ie a 'junior' aspirin) a day. Warfarin or other anticoagulants (clot-preventing drugs) are sometimes used if there is a risk of a blood clot forming in the heart (eg in some people with an altered heart rhythm known as **atrial fibrilation**).

The cause of a stroke must be correctly diagnosed before aspirin and anticoagulants are prescribed. If the cause is haemorrhage (bleeding) into the brain, anticoagulants are not recommended. Haemorrhage can usually be detected by a CT scan (see p 22) of the head.

Removing blockages in the carotid artery

An operation (carotid endarterectomy) may be offered to someone who has had a TIA or minor stroke caused by a narrowing (stenosis) of the carotid artery. In cases of severe carotid blockage the surgical removal of the blockage can reduce the risk of stroke by between six and ten times. But there is a very slight risk; between 2 and 4 per cent of patients may die or have a major stroke within 30 days of the operation. Someone who is thought to need this operation should be referred to a specialist in cerebrovascular disease (disease of the brain and its blood vessels). The specialist (who could be a neurologist, vascular surgeon or physician) can establish that the cause of the TIA or stroke lies in the narrowing of the carotid artery. Ask the doctor to explain the benefits and risks of investigation or surgery, and the alternatives.

The stages of stroke and recovery

Although stroke affects everyone differently, there is a common pattern to the way in which people recover and rebuild their lives. Understanding this pattern may help you plan for the future.

Stroke and immediate care

A stroke can occur at any time or place, and usually develops suddenly, but sometimes over a number of hours. In about 50 per cent of people, the stroke reaches its full extent within 6 hours, and 19 out of 20 people will be over the worst in 24 hours. Most people who are going to die from a serious stroke do so during the first day.

In the early stages, first aid is needed to protect the person from falling over and hurting himself as a result of paralysis, or from choking or suffocating if he is unconscious. It may be relatives, bystanders or, later, the GP, ambulance crew or hospital who give this care. At the present time there is usually little that can be done in this stage to limit the impact of the stroke, so it may be difficult to decide whether your relative should stay at home or go into hospital. At home, the person is in familiar surroundings, attended by his GP and cared for by his relatives. In hospital there is the option of tests to diagnose the type of stroke and, in some cases, the possibility that doctors can intervene in some way. But in most cases the care is the same: stabilising the patient and preventing him coming to further harm. Your decision also has implications for future care, treatment and support, and you may find it helpful to read the next chapter which discusses this more fully.

Recovery

Recovery usually takes place naturally but, without good care, many physical, social and psychological complications can occur which greatly limit recovery. During a stroke some brain cells die and others remain alive but temporarily stop working because of a lack of blood. The dead cells swell and put pressure on other cells, which also stop working. Recovery happens when an adequate blood supply is restored to cells that had a meagre supply, and, when the swelling goes down, allowing the cells under pressure to start working normally again. As the cells 'come on line', the abilities they control are restored. This usually happens within two or three weeks, but it varies from person to person. As well as this short-term, sometimes spectacular, recovery there is usually a more gradual recovery. This takes place over years, as undamaged cells take over some of the jobs of cells that have died, and as new pathways develop to carry messages within the brain and between the brain and the muscles.

Rehabilitation

Rehabilitation is the process of learning to overcome a disability. It involves learning changes in approach, behaviour and the use of muscles. Depending on your relative's needs, a physiotherapist, occupational therapist and/or speech and language therapist can offer advice and training on ways of overcoming different disabilities. Unless there are complications, rehabilitation should start in the early stages of the stroke. The longer a person remains inactive, the more work it takes to regain mobility. Although rehabilitation starts in hospital, much will take place at home. Regaining independence takes persistence and dedication by the person who has had the stroke, and by those who care for him. It is often a slow process but much can be achieved. Hope for the future is soundly based: 65 per cent of those who cannot walk unaided immediately after a stroke will eventually be able to walk alone, and within six months of a stroke 90 per cent of people are fully continent.

Adaptation

Sometimes adapting the environment can help to restore independence. This might be something as simple as using a walking stick, or it might involve structural alterations to a building or vehicle to help your relative get about. In between are a whole range of devices and adaptations to make life easier. You and your relative will also need to make a psychological adaptation to the new circumstances and to what is possible in the future. You may both have to consider changes in your occupation, living arrangements or social life, and even in your attitudes and aspirations.

Independence/long-term care

Progress often continues for up to two years and beyond, but after about six months you should have a good idea of your relative's future care needs. About 30 per cent of people are able to return to a fairly normal life after a stroke, but about 50 per cent have some residual mental or physical disability. The amount of care needed varies enormously from person to person – some will never be able to return home and will go into a care home but many will show no outward sign of any problem. Remember that having a disability is not the same thing as being dependent. Most people regain the ability to get out of bed, get dressed and walk unaided, and about half regain the ability to feed themselves. By working out where support is essential, and where skills can be developed, it may be possible for your relative to achieve a good degree of independence.

Encouraging independence in your relative right from the start can help to make life easier for both of you in the long term. Perhaps surprisingly, the quickest and most complete recovery seems to take place among the 20 per cent of people who go home to live alone, because they *have* to learn to do things for themselves.

Helping your relative develop independence requires sensitivity, patience and, sometimes, emotional toughness, but is well worth the effort. You may want to help whenever your relative finds something difficult, but it is important not to undermine his self-confidence or deny him the opportunity to learn. You need to find a balance: give plenty of support, but avoid creating long-term dependence which you might both come to regret.

For more *i*nformation

ⓘ *Stroke: a self-help manual for stroke sufferers and their families* by Dr RM Youngson, published by David and Charles.

ⓘ *Stroke: a practical guide towards recovery* by Dr R Langton Hewer and Dr DT Wade, published by Vermilion.

ⓘ *Living with Stroke* by Paul King, published by Manchester University Press. (This book is out of print, but may be available in libraries.)

ⓘ *Practical Management of Stroke* by Dr GP Mulley, published by Chapman and Hall, London, 1988.

ⓘ Stroke Association publications:

Booklet S5 *Understanding stroke illness*

Booklet S7 *Stroke – a handbook for the patient's family*

Leaflet S3 *Reducing the risk of a stroke*

Leaflet S11 *What is a TIA?*

Leaflet S12 *Facts about high blood pressure*

Leaflet SF11 *High blood pressure? Why you need to take your drugs*

2 What to do when your relative has a stroke

The early days after someone has had a stroke are likely to be stressful. There is the initial shock; the immediate need to get medical help; worry about whether to keep the ill person at home or send her to hospital; anxiety about the development of the stroke and the future outlook; concern about the quality of treatment your relative is getting; and perhaps the need to rearrange your life so you can care for your relative at home or visit her in hospital.

This chapter is designed to help you in those early days. It gives advice on caring for someone immediately after a stroke. It suggests the factors you should consider when deciding whether your relative could stay at home or should go into hospital. And it describes the sorts of treatment she is likely to receive. Finally it discusses the likelihood of recovery and survival.

Sean

'The doctor said May should go into hospital, but May was adamant she wanted to stay at home'

'I didn't know what to do for the best. To keep May at home or send for an ambulance.

17

'May got down to clean the stove and found she couldn't stand up. I helped her into the hall but I couldn't move her any further; she's heavier than me. I managed to reach the phone and called the doctor. Our son arrived and we moved her on to the settee. The doctor said May should go into hospital, but May was adamant she wanted to stay at home. Later on, when she lost consciousness, I phoned for an ambulance. We had to wait for hours before anyone saw us at the hospital.'

Recognising a stroke

The symptoms of stroke vary enormously but often involve weakness or paralysis of the face, arm or leg, and some loss of speech. About one-third of people remain fully conscious throughout, another third become confused, and the final third become unconscious. Other common effects are difficulty in swallowing (in about a third of cases) and changes in the sense of touch or feeling (in about a quarter of cases).

A stroke can happen anywhere and at any time, but most occur at home. About one in five people has a stroke while they are asleep. Most people can tell you what is happening to them, but about a third lose the ability to speak. About one in twenty people has a fit (convulsion).

What to do when someone has a stroke

Always give first aid first. Then get medical help.

■ Give first aid to ensure physical safety. If the person is unconscious, make sure that she does not choke. Put her in the first aid 'recovery' position. If you don't know how to do this, put the person on her side and tilt her head backwards. Make sure that her mouth is pointing downwards so that she cannot choke on her tongue or on her vomit if she is sick. Do not leave the person on her back.

■ Be careful not to pull on a paralysed limb. Pulling or falling on to a paralysed limb can damage muscle, bones or joints. Hold and move her by her trunk.

■ If your relative is unconscious and you can't move her on to her side, get help immediately from a passer-by or neighbours.

■ If the person has a fit, clear space around her. Move or cover furniture and sharp objects with cushions to prevent injury. Don't try to put anything in her mouth or to remove dentures forcibly.

■ If the person is conscious, make her comfortable, again taking care not to move her by a paralysed arm or leg.

■ Phone an ambulance or the person's GP.

Whether to call an ambulance or the GP

Although doctors can do little in the first stages to limit the extent of the stroke or speed the recovery, they *can* help the recovery process and prevent further complications. The decision whether to call an ambulance or to call the GP is a complicated one. It depends on:

■ the seriousness of the stroke;

■ your ability to provide care at home;

■ your confidence in the GP.

Bear in mind that the long-term outcome *is* significantly affected by the quality of care and advice your relative receives in the early days. Both hospitals and GPs act as gatekeepers to the other services that your relative needs to recover. These services vary widely. Some hospitals have specialist stroke wards or rehabilitation wards. In others, a stroke patient may be placed in a general ward, geriatric ward, cardiac ward or neurological ward.

Seriousness of the stroke

Your relative should go into hospital if:

■ she is unconscious and you are unable to prevent her from choking;

■ she has had a fit lasting more than two minutes;

- the doctor is not sure of the diagnosis and further tests need to be done;
- there is no one to care for her at home.

Going into hospital could also be beneficial if the person is paralysed or has difficulties in speaking. Stroke patients need well-planned, careful and skilled care from an early stage to achieve maximum recovery, and it may be easier to arrange this in hospital. Rest is *not* the best thing. Older people quickly lose muscle bulk and strength. For each week spent resting in bed, one-tenth of the remaining muscular strength is lost, and recovering it requires long, hard work.

In hospital, physiotherapists may encourage your relative to start moving the day after she has had her stroke. They will protect paralysed limbs, re-teach movement and prevent bad habits being formed right from the start. Speech therapists can make an early assessment of your relative's swallowing as well as language problems and advise you both on how to tackle them.

If you care for your relative at home, the GP will arrange the nursing and therapy she needs.

Your ability to provide care at home

Before you decide whether to keep your relative at home, you need to think about how you will care for her:

- Do you feel confident about giving nursing care? Have you got the physical strength that this may need?
- How much time will caring take up, and for how long?
- What will the costs of caring be? Will you need to take time off work?
- What support can you expect from professional carers, other relatives and friends?
- How will you cope with someone who is unconscious, incontinent or who may die?
- If you do not live with your relative, can you provide adequate care from a distance?
- How will you travel to hospital? How much time will travelling and visiting take?

■ What about your other commitments? The needs of your family, perhaps, or your job?

Your confidence in your relative's GP

If you choose to keep your relative at home, the GP will play a crucial role in her care. The GP will diagnose and treat your relative, but is also the key to arranging other care services that will help her recover: for example, access to a speech and language therapist, occupational therapist and/or physiotherapist; access to nursing care from the district nurse or community psychiatric nurse; and access to help from social services. A good GP can also put you in touch with voluntary support agencies such as Age Concern and the Stroke Association.

It is important that you feel confident in the GP. It is worth bearing in mind that the average GP sees only four or five stroke patients each year, whereas a general hospital serving a population of 250,000 is likely to see 500 cases every year. In the Stroke Association survey *A Voice for Stroke*, 60 per cent of respondents felt they had not been adequately advised and supported by their GP, and gave a lack of information as the main reason for problems. If you are not confident in the GP, you may want to consider changing doctor.

If you do opt for home care in the early stages, you need to think carefully about what this may involve. For example:

■ Tasks demanding physical strength, such as helping someone to get out of bed, to walk or to turn over in bed.
■ Practical nursing tasks such as turning your relative to prevent pressure (bed) sores, helping her to use the toilet, bathing her.
■ Learning the correct way to help someone who is paralysed to sit up, get out of bed and walk.
■ Negotiating the range of health services that your relative will need, such as physiotherapy, occupational therapy, speech therapy.
■ Helping your relative to learn and practise techniques to regain movement, balance or speech.

- Contacting social services and other agencies to get the help and support that you need.
- Giving your relative a great deal of encouragement and emotional support.
- Coping with your own feelings about caring for someone and the changes that this will bring to your life.

Which professionals can help?

Caring for your relative calls on the skills of different professionals. Some provide services in hospital, some provide help for people at home, and some do both. Services and job titles vary from area to area, but the list on pages 44–47 describes the professionals you are most likely to meet, and the help they can provide. Your relative's GP is likely to play a crucial role. He or she can provide access to a range of community-based health services and can refer your relative to hospital services or to a hospital consultant. If you think your relative needs professional help but it isn't offered, always ask for it.

Diagnostic tests

Normally diagnosis is confirmed through the doctor taking a detailed history. But in about one in twenty cases the diagnosis is not straightforward. Your doctor may also need to rule out cerebral haemorrhage as the cause of the stroke before prescribing anticoagulant drugs (see p 12). In these cases various tests may be done; some of the common ones are described below.

A **CT** (computed tomography) **scan** takes X-ray pictures of the brain and can identify other conditions that mimic stroke but may require quite different treatment.

An **ECG** (electrocardiogram) is a record of electrical impulses from the heart; it can identify problems in the heart.

A **blood sample** can be tested for high levels of cholesterol; high levels of blood sugar, which may indicate diabetes; and a higher than average tendency for the blood to clot.

If a blockage in the carotid artery is suspected, two techniques are commonly used:

An **ultra-sound scan** can predict the presence or absence of a narrowing of the artery (stenosis: see Glossary). The scan carries no additional risk to the patient.

A **carotid angiogram** involves injecting a dye either directly into the carotid artery or inserting a long needle into one of the arteries of the legs. X-rays are taken of the neck, and the dye clearly reveals the presence of any blockages. Ask the consultant, or one of the doctors in the consultant's team, for more information about the benefits, risks and alternatives to this investigation in your relative's case.

What are the chances of survival?

If the stroke is very severe, and the ill person becomes unconscious, incontinent or is severely paralysed, there is a possibility that she may die. Someone with these symptoms is at greatest risk of dying on the first day and, sadly, about a third of people who have a stroke die within three weeks.

But the way that stroke affects people varies enormously, so it is impossible to predict exactly what will happen. Talk to your relative's doctor. He or she is the best person to give you an honest assessment of the likely outcome.

There is evidence that people who *regain* control over their bladder within about three days are likely to make a good recovery in terms of walking and getting home. In their book *Stroke*, Richard Langton Hewer and Derek Wade explain the chances of recovery based on other symptoms of patients at their hospital in Bristol:

- Someone who is unable to walk unaided immediately after a stroke has a 65 per cent chance of being able to walk alone.
- Someone who cannot dress alone immediately after a stroke has a 67 per cent chance of being able to do so.

■ Someone who cannot eat without help after a stroke has a 54 per cent chance of being able to do so.

■ Someone who cannot get out of bed into a chair without help, has a 68 per cent chance of being able to do so.

■ Someone whose arm has no movement after two weeks has a 40 per cent chance of regaining the use of that arm.

Although these statistics seem rather gloomy, recovery can be helped by the determination of the person who has had a stroke, and the encouragement she gets from those around her. At six months after a stroke most people are continent and can use the toilet, wash, bathe, shave and dress themselves with little or no help; eat without help; get out of bed; walk and use the stairs. *Stroke News*, the quarterly magazine of the Stroke Association, regularly features the stories of people who have suffered severe strokes and have made remarkable recoveries.

For more *i*nformation

i *Stroke: a practical guide* by Dr RL Hewer and Dr DT Wade, published by Vermilion.

i Stroke Association publications:

Booklet S5 *Understanding stroke illness*

Booklet S7 *Stroke – a handbook for the patient's family*

Leaflet S17 *What is carotid endarterectomy?*

3 The effects of stroke

To hear that your relative has had a stroke tells you little about the problems that he is likely to face or the disabilities that he will have to overcome. Before you can start to assess how the stroke will affect your lives, you need to know more about the site of the stroke, the extent of the stroke and how the brain is organised to carry out different tasks.

This chapter explains how the brain is organised into specialised areas and describes some of the more common effects of stroke. It also explains some of the medical terms you are likely to hear.

Kulbinda

'It's helped him a lot working in the shop.'

'Ranjit can still speak and understand Punjabi, but he can no longer speak English. He works in the shop though he can't carry the heavier things like rolls of cable. He operates the till with his left hand and gets on great; if anyone can't speak Punjabi he calls Harinder. It's helped him a lot working in the shop; he was a little miserable before he got back there, but now it helps him in so many ways.'

A general understanding of the brain and how it communicates with the muscles will help you to understand how damage to the brain causes your relative's problems. With this understanding you will be able to have more fruitful discussions with the doctors and therapists and will avoid expecting more of your relative than he is capable of.

Activities such as talking and seeing are not simple abilities which you either do or do not have; they depend on many different parts of the brain working together. After a stroke some of these parts may be missing, causing gaps in abilities which are not immediately evident. If you are unaware of this it is easy to think that your relative is being deliberately stubborn or lazy, when in fact he has not understood or cannot do what you are asking of him.

The brain and the nervous system

The brain is the centre of the body's nervous system, which gathers information, processes it and gives instructions to the muscles. The brain has the central role of analysing information and sending instructions. It is connected to the rest of the body by the spinal cord, which runs down the length of the spine. A network of nerves spreads out from the spinal column to connect the brain to the rest of the body.

Besides carrying information to and from the brain, the spinal cord sends some instructions to the muscles direct. In an undamaged brain these messages are monitored and regulated by the brain. When stroke damages the brain this control function is sometimes lost, causing the muscles to contract and stay shortened in the weak limbs ('spasticity': see Glossary).

The brain has three main parts:

The **cerebrum**: this is the top and largest part of the brain; it is divided into two halves called the left and the right hemispheres.

The **cerebellum**: this lies at the back of the brain, under the cerebrum and behind the brain stem.

The **brain stem**: this lies at the bottom of the brain and connects the brain to the spinal cord.

The outer layer of the cerebrum is called the cerebral cortex. This is where many important brain functions are carried out. Nerves pass from the cortex through the centre of the brain and down the brain stem to connect the cortex with the rest of the body. A stroke in the centre of the brain or in the brain stem will have far-reaching effects because it damages these connections to the cortex.

The division of the brain into two hemispheres is important because each side performs different tasks. Strokes tend to occur on one side or the other, limiting the functions on that side.

Each hemisphere is divided into four lobes:

The **frontal lobe** is at the front of the brain.

The **parietal lobe** is in the middle, top part of the brain behind the frontal lobe.

The **temporal lobe** is at the side of the brain below the parietal lobe.

The **occipital lobe** is at the back of the brain.

Map of the main areas of the brain

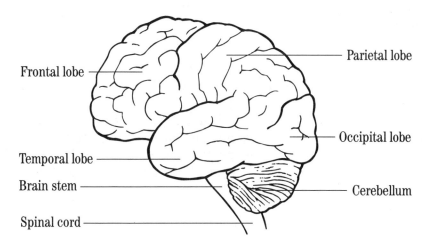

27

What different parts of the brain do

For most people the left temporal lobe controls language and the right temporal lobe the sense of space. In a very small number of people these positions are reversed. The occipital lobe makes sense of visual input – what a person sees.

Each hemisphere controls the movement on the opposite side of the body. The nerves from the left side cross over in the brain stem and spinal cord to control the right side of the body, and the nerves from the right side cross over to control the left side of the body. This is why a stroke in the left hemisphere causes paralysis of the right side of the body and a stroke in the right hemisphere affects the left side of the body. And it is why speech difficulties are usually associated with right-sided paralysis and difficulties in making sense of the left side of space or of one's body with left-sided paralysis.

Another important split into halves occurs with eyesight. The nerves connecting the eye to the brain split what is seen by each eye into left and right halves. The messages from the left half of both eyes go to one side of the occipital lobe and the messages from the right half of both eyes to the other side of the occipital lobe. This means that, if the part of the brain that controls the left side of vision is affected by a stroke, all sight is lost on the left side; similarly, if the stroke affects the part controlling right-sided vision, all sight is lost on the right.

This is called **hemianopia**, which comes from the Greek *hemi* meaning half, *an* meaning without and *opia* meaning vision. Sufferers of hemianopia lose sight completely on one side. Often they are unaware that they have lost their sight on the one side, and this causes them to ignore anything on that side. So they will not realise that someone is standing on their blind side and they will ignore conversation from that side. They may not see objects on their blind side and may bump into things placed on that side.

Map of the different brain functions

This map of the brain shows the layout of function for most people. In a small number of cases – eg in some people who are naturally left-handed – the right and left functions are swapped over and so, for example, the language centre is on the right-hand side.

Left

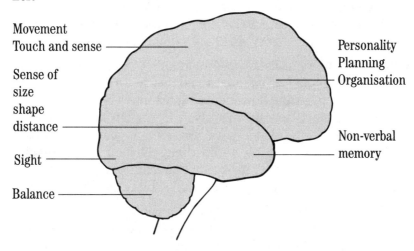

Movement
Touch and sense

Sense of
size
shape
distance

Sight

Balance

Personality
Planning
Organisation

Non-verbal
memory

Right

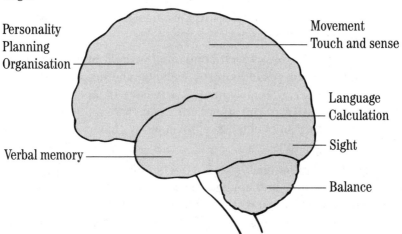

Personality
Planning
Organisation

Verbal memory

Movement
Touch and sense

Language
Calculation

Sight

Balance

The effects of stroke damage to different areas of the brain

Looking at the brain map we can see the effects of stroke in different areas. A stroke on the left-hand side of the brain could affect language and movement and the sense of feeling on the right side – including the face, arm and leg. People with right-sided weakness are often slow and clumsy and have communication difficulties.

A stroke on the right-hand side could affect the area of brain that gives understanding of distances and space, so activities such as washing, eating, sitting down, pouring tea into a cup become more difficult. It could also cause paralysis of the left-hand side of the body. People with left-sided paralysis often appear to be unaware of their limitations and try to do things beyond their capability. Because they can speak and communicate well, other people sometimes under-estimate how much disability they have suffered.

Strokes in the occipital lobe damage vision, and strokes in the brain stem can sometimes be fatal because the brain stem controls basic bodily functions such as breathing and circulation. Co-ordination and balance are affected by strokes in the cerebellum.

Paralysis (loss of power) of one side of the body is called **hemiplegia**, and incomplete paralysis is called **hemiparesis**. Paralysis is common because so much of the brain is involved in movement. Areas involved in movement are:

■ both parietal lobes, which control movement and sensation;
■ the cerebellum, which controls balance and co-ordination;
■ the pyramidal system, which is a cluster of nerves that connects the cortex to the spinal cord and carries the instructions for voluntary movements (movements that you choose to make) to the muscles.

Damage to the pyramidal system affects movement even when the parietal lobes are undamaged because it breaks the lines of communication between the movement areas of the brain and the muscles. Fortunately, there is another system of nerve connections, mainly concerned with involuntary muscular action (movement that happens automatically), which can to a limited extent take over functions performed by the pyramidal system. This is what seems to happen when recovery takes place.

Nerves from the surface areas of the brain pass through the brain, come together, connect to the brain stem and run on to form the spinal cord. A stroke at any of these points can cause disabilities.

Even simple activities depend on many parts of the brain working together. Think, for example, of the different abilities involved if you say to someone 'Go out of the door and turn left':

- hearing
- language and understanding
- memory
- ability to make voluntary leg movements
- the ability to see or feel
- co-ordination and balance
- recognition of objects
- knowing what left and right mean

These abilities are built up from more specialised brain functions, any one of which might be damaged by a stroke.

The problems faced by someone who has had a stroke are looked at below in four areas:

- Physical problems
- Sensory problems
- Psychological and emotional problems
- Problems with understanding

Physical problems

Paralysis

Weakness, paralysis and a loss of feeling are common after stroke. They can affect any part of the body but are most obvious when they affect the face, arm and leg. The loss of control varies from clumsiness and tremor to full paralysis. Even when physical strength and the ability to move are undamaged, your relative may still be unable to walk because a stroke in the cerebellum affects his sense of balance and co-ordination. Similarly, simple activities like making a cup of tea may be beyond your relative, not because his muscles have been affected but because he can no longer remember how to do things – this special type of loss is to do with difficulty in starting the movements and doing them in the right order (**apraxia**) and has important consequences for speech and writing.

Secondary problems of paralysis

Paralysis can lead to other problems if it is not treated correctly from the start. These are:

- pressure sores
- blood clots in the lung
- chest infections
- constipation
- 'frozen' shoulder
- spasticity

Lack of movement can result in pressure sores, chest infections and constipation. It can also cause blood clots to form in the leg, which then move up to the lungs to cause a pulmonary embolism. 'Frozen' shoulder is caused by the mishandling of someone with a paralysed arm. Spasticity happens when the spinal cord instructs muscles to tense and this can no longer be overriden by the brain because it or the connecting nerves are damaged. The muscles go into spasm (tension), and if nothing is done about it they will freeze in this position. This may limit further recovery and reha- bilitation. Correct positioning of the limbs can reduce the risk of this happening.

Swallowing difficulties

Swallowing involves many different muscles and nerves. Problems with any of these can cause swallowing difficulties. This can cause hunger and discomfort; constipation because of insufficient fluid intake; and could lead to a chest infection because food and other items pass into the windpipe.

Incontinence

Incontinence of both the bladder and the bowels is a common consequence of stroke. For most people incontinence clears up rapidly.

Sensory problems

Loss or weakening of the senses of touch and sight are common consequences of stroke; damage to taste, smell and hearing are less common.

Touch

Change to the sense of touch varies: with some people it is a loss of sensitivity such that differences in texture can no longer be felt; with others just a gentle touch can be painful.

Eyesight

The commonest effect is 'half-blindness', or hemianopia. With hemianopia, performing simple tasks becomes very difficult because half the picture is missing. If your relative suffers from this he may bump into objects or people and fail to respond to hazards on his blind side. For most people hemianopia is not permanent but, for the small number who are left with permanent hemianopia, training can help to develop awareness of the blind side.

Psychological and emotional problems

Stroke may cause rapid mood shifts in your relative and change aspects of his character. Depression is a common experience after stroke although how much of it is caused by the stroke and how much of it is a natural response to the life changes caused by the stroke is not clear. Sudden switching of moods into laughing or weeping for apparently trivial reasons is called emotional lability; it usually settles down after a few months. Sometimes the scarring of brain tissue can cause fits to develop after a stroke. These can usually be controlled by medication.

There may be problems with continuing a sexual relationship after stroke. The problems may be physical, psychological or caused by medicines. In a small number of cases, a stroke can affect a person's previous learning such that he may lose his inhibitions about what is and isn't appropriate sexual behaviour. This can be embarrassing or distressing for those around him. It helps to remember that the person is not aware there is anything inappropriate or wrong in what he is doing – it is the stroke that causes him to behave in this way. Although this can be a difficult subject to talk about, doctors and nurses who work with stroke patients will understand and can offer practical help and support. Talk to your GP or someone from the psychiatric support team. For more information about sexual relationships after a stroke, see pages 89–90.

Emotional and psychological problems are dealt with in Chapter 7.

Problems with understanding

Memory

This is often affected by stroke. Memory is not located in one part of the brain but is split into different sorts of memories for different activities; for example, there is a visual memory and there is a language memory. Part of the memory can remain while other parts are impaired.

Our memories appear to be ordered into three layers: an immediate memory, a mid-term memory and a long-term memory. The immediate memory holds things that have happened in the last few seconds, the mid-term memory allows us to recall events from beyond a few moments ago and into the recent past, and the long-term memory allows recall from beyond the recent past. Learning has to pass through the mid-term memory before it goes into the long-term memory. Unfortunately for many people who have had a stroke, it is the mid-term memory that is usually damaged. Immediate events and events from long ago can be recalled but not, for example, what was learnt at the last therapy session. This makes learning, and therefore rehabilitation, difficult.

Understanding

Understanding is sometimes affected by stroke, either partially or completely. When understanding is only partially affected it becomes apparent in inappropriate responses to conversation or situations. Damage to understanding that is not immediately obvious sometimes arises with strokes to the right hemisphere. These damage the person's perception of space and so relations like inside/outside, top/bottom and near/far are no longer clearly understood.

It is important not to make assumptions though. Many people who are unable to speak have their understanding fully intact and it is a cause of great distress to them that other people assume that it is not.

Concentration

Concentration can also be affected. This makes skilled tasks difficult because of lapses of attention. It also makes learning difficult. Everyday activities that are potentially dangerous, such as cooking with boiling water or using matches to light a gas appliance, can no longer be carried out.

Speech

The loss of speech is one of the most distressing outcomes of stroke. It can cause despair to both the person who has had the stroke and his family. It is, however, fairly rare to lose completely the ability to communicate.

Most people have their speech centres on the left side of their brain. Damage to this side affects speech, understanding, reading and writing. Speech has two elements:

- the ability to express speech;
- the ability to understand speech.

Damage may occur to one element and not the other. It is quite common for speech to be affected but not understanding. To help understand difficulties with speech and language, it is useful to look at what happens when we speak. It involves four stages:

- the idea
- translating the idea into the word
- remembering how to say (or write) the word
- moving the appropriate muscles to make the required sounds (or write the required words).

These functions are performed by different parts of the brain. Speech can be affected when any one of these functions is damaged.

Speech and language therapists and doctors identify three different types of speech disorder: apraxia, aphasia and dysarthria.

Aphasia

This is the inability to translate ideas into words. People suffering from aphasia may not speak at all or may use inappropriate words. The amount of aphasia varies (less than full aphasia is sometimes called dysphasia). It affects both understanding and the expression of speech, although they do not necessarily occur together. People suffering from mild aphasia lose subtle meanings of words or occasionally lose the meaning of a sentence or two.

Apraxia

This is the inability to start or put in the right order the muscle movements necessary to make a word. In someone suffering from apraxia, odd sounds often appear in the middle of their words. The ability to understand is not affected. Speech may be affected where writing is not, or vice versa. In writing, words may be spelled wrongly or letters not formed properly. Dyspraxia is the milder form of apraxia.

Dysarthia

This occurs when the muscles that produce speech – those that control breathing, the throat, palate, tongue and lips – are affected. Only pronunciation is affected. Understanding and the choice of words and how to say them are not. Dysarthia may occur after a stroke affecting one of the cerebral hemispheres or the brain stem. If eyesight and arm movements are not damaged, reading and writing are not affected by dysarthria.

Other causes of difficulty in reading and writing

Stroke causes many sight problems, which may affect the ability to read and write. Hemianopia makes it difficult to read because half the words on the page are not visible. Damage to the perception of space may also make writing and reading difficult.

The social consequences of stroke

Stroke can have important social consequences, both for the person who has the stroke and for those who care for him. They might include:

- a change in the relationship between you and your relative;
- a change in the relationship between your relative and the rest of the family;
- ending of work for you and your relative;
- a substantial change in income;
- restrictions on continuing old social activities such as helping at church, politics, involvement in societies, sports and leisure;
- loss of friends because activities can no longer be shared;
- reduced mobility for you and your relative;
- social avoidance by your relative because of difficulty in talking;
- no independent time for you because of the needs of your relative;
- reduced opportunities for socialising because money is short.

Although stroke can have significant social effects, it doesn't have to. There are many examples of people who have suffered severe strokes and have rebuilt fulfilling lives. Most people make remarkable recoveries and good rehabilitation minimises the effects of disability. Support is available from the health services, the local authority and the voluntary sector. New opportunities for socialising open as the old ones close down. Respite care enables carers to maintain a regular social life of their own and still provide the best care for their relative.

The social effects of stroke depend to some extent on the person's commitments before the stroke. If someone is relatively young, the effect on employment is a major concern. If he also has a young family, the effect on the family relationships and circumstances will have to be taken into account when planning for the future. (See also pp 88 and 120.)

The disabilities caused by stroke and the need for care do impose restrictions on social activities but, by making use of the advice and support organisations listed in this book, you and your relative should be able to find your own way to a full and rewarding social life.

For more *i*nformation

ⓘ *Stroke: A practical guide towards recovery* by Dr RL Hewer and Dr DT Wade, published by Vermilion.

ⓘ *Living with Stroke* by Paul King, published by Manchester University Press. Out of print but may be available at your local library.

ⓘ Stroke Association booklets:

S5 *Understanding stroke illness*

S7 *Stroke – a handbook for the patient's family*

S25 *Cognitive problems following stroke*

4 What can be done?

Assessing an individual's likely recovery is extremely difficult. It depends on the extent and location of the stroke, the individual's motivation, and the support of family and friends. Even so, results vary enormously. Some people make almost complete recoveries, whereas others still have considerable mental impairment one year later. The quality of care and support can make a substantial difference to the outcome. This chapter looks at the services available to help your relative recover and at what you can do to help.

Ella

'She worked intensively with him five days a week, and that's how he can talk.'

'Without Sophie, the speech therapist, Trevor wouldn't be talking.

'Trevor had a severe right-sided stroke; it was three months before he could say anything. He was back at the counter at the post office for six months, but couldn't speak. Then Sophie took an interest in his case. She worked intensively with him for five days a week, and that's how he can talk. Ask him yourself – she transformed his life.'

Recovery

How well do people recover?

Some people make astonishing recoveries from stroke. (See pp 23–24 for more information about recovery rates.) Much recovery takes place spontaneously, but constant encouragement and the appropriate help of therapists will enable your relative to build on this as well. The person's will to recover can also be important, and you can help by taking every opportunity to nurture this.

About half the people who have a stroke survive the first year. Of these, 85 per cent will survive the next year, and so on for subsequent years. Most survivors of stroke do not die from stroke but from heart disease or some other cause.

It is the site not the size of the damage to the brain that determines the likely outcome. Damage to the central brain is more serious than damage to the cortex. People with perceptual and visual problems, especially hemianopia (see p 28), often experience greater difficulty in relearning daily activities. Generally, recovery of walking ability is better than recovery of the use of the hand and arm.

A severe stroke may have worse long-term effects and recovery may be slower. Long-held skills are generally retained better than newly learned ones. Treatment should start early for fullest recovery of language and of physical skills such as walking and arm movements. Many people, even the elderly, make a relatively good recovery. One in ten people appears to have no loss of ability at all.

How long does it take to recover abilities?

Recovery is most rapid in the first three months; by six months most recovery has been achieved. But with the right encouragement and therapies there are plenty of examples of remarkable recoveries after this period. Between six months and two years there is usually some slow, steady progress. After two years it is unusual for further recovery to occur. With all abilities – memory, walking, strength, language – an early recovery indicates better prospects for full recovery. If full movement is going to return to the arm, for example, some voluntary movement of the arm will occur within the first two weeks. Language shows a similar pattern. See page 42 for more information.

How can therapy help?

Therapy can:

■ Prevent complications such as frozen shoulder or spasticity.

■ Help the person to adapt and use remaining abilities to overcome disabilities; for example, a skilled physiotherapist can help someone to walk.

■ Help to retrain the brain and prevent it learning non-use. When the brain tries to use a limb and cannot, it may, after a number of attempts, simply give up trying. Techniques to encourage even the slightest movements in limbs can prevent this.

There is more detailed information on page 44 about the ways in which different therapists can help. It makes a big difference if everyone helps, not just the trained therapist. A therapist can diagnose the problems, recommend the best way to tackle them, and train the person with a stroke and her carers to use exercises and techniques designed to help recovery. If you can, get involved from the start in meetings with the therapist, especially if the stroke has affected your relative's ability to concentrate.

The pattern of recovery

Although individuals vary, there is often a common pattern of recovery for someone who is bedridden after a stroke. Abilities are likely to return in this order:

■ Sitting in a chair and eating food that has been already cut up.

■ Continence – bowel before bladder.

■ Walking with assistance.

■ Washing, shaving, cleaning teeth, etc.

■ Dressing with help.

■ Getting out of bed and walking unaided.

■ Eating unaided.

■ Using stairs without help.
■ Using the bath without help.

Your relative's progress will depend on the severity of the stroke and on what she could do before; an older person who had difficulty using the bath before a stroke, for example, may well have greater difficulty afterwards.

Speech

About 60 per cent of stroke sufferers have minor problems with speech in the first few days. About one in ten loses the ability to speak at all; this is caused by damage to one of the speech centres. A third of people with right-sided weakness have language disturbance, but those with left-sided weakness rarely have problems. Language ability usually improves most in the early weeks and less as time goes on.

Recovering use of a leg

Recovery from paralysis usually begins with the return of control of the leg: 80 per cent of stroke survivors will walk again. Good quality rehabilitation makes a significant difference: for example, patients in stroke units tend to recover more mobility than patients in general wards. A quarter of the survivors of a first stroke recover their previous walking ability, but predicting who will and who will not make a good recovery is difficult, especially in the first ten weeks.

Recovering use of an arm

Stroke has the most serious and long-lasting effects on the most delicate movements. The face and hand, for example, often fail to recover their previous mobility. In the arm, movement returns first to the shoulder, then the elbow and finally the wrist and fingers. The ability to straighten the arm, wrist or fingers returns after the ability to bend them. In people who have a paralysed side after a stroke, 15 per cent will lose the ability to move their arm, 40 per cent will regain some movement and 45 per cent will gain full voluntary movement of the arm but not necessarily fine movements of the hand.

How you can help recovery

Helping your relative to recover her abilities will inevitably make demands on your time and on your emotions. You will have to provide support without encouraging dependence and this will need a sensitive balance between sympathy and firmness.

Give your relative emotional and practical support Support her motivation to get better. You can help by organising the right type of support, creating a stimulating environment, keeping up social contacts and, if necessary, dealing on your relative's behalf with the professionals. But most of all you need to show her that she is still valued as a person and has an important place in family life.

Work in partnership with the therapists Make sure your relative gets a proper assessment and accurate diagnosis of her difficulties from the appropriate therapist. If you can, learn the exercises and support activities along with your relative so that you can help her continue them at home. Help her get into a routine to do them regularly.

Give your relative frequent encouragement Even if you don't live with your relative, you can still do a lot to provide the kinds of emotional and practical help suggested here.

Rehabilitation

The aim of rehabilitation is to help people to reach their full potential and make the most of the abilities that they have. So rehabilitation tries to *extend* the abilities that recover spontaneously and to prevent complications that might limit the degree of recovery. The consultant in hospital and the GP in the community have a key role in this process, co-ordinating the activities of other specialists.

Rehabilitation may involve physiotherapy, occupational therapy and/or speech therapy, and the help of other professionals such as a hospital liaison nurse, a social worker, a district nurse and a community psychiatric nurse. The ward nurse is a key person in rehabilitation while your relative is recovering in hospital. In some areas professionals involved in rehabilitation work closely in a well-organised team. In other areas the rehabilitation team is less well co-ordinated, and services are more patchy.

Who does what?

The consultant

If your relative goes into hospital, or is referred by her GP to an out-patients' clinic, she will be under the care of a consultant. A consultant specialises in a particular area of medicine and may develop areas of special interest. A general physician, for example, may develop a special interest in stroke. (Ask the hospital liaison worker if there is a consultant who specialises in stroke.)

- a general physician provides general medical care but often has a specialism as well;
- a cardiologist specialises in heart disease;
- a geriatrician specialises in treating older people;
- a neurologist treats diseases of the brain and nervous system;
- a psychiatrist treats psychological and mental health problems;
- a psychogeriatrician specialises in mental illnesses in older people (eg dementia, depression);
- a consultant in stroke medicine (only in some hospitals) specialises in treating people who have had a stroke.

Therapists

Most physiotherapists, occupational therapists and speech therapists work with people in hospital, but a growing number work with people in their home. Some do both.

The physiotherapist

The physiotherapist can help someone with a stroke to overcome paralysis, regain movement in the limbs and body, and improve balance. Ideally, your relative should see a physiotherapist from the first day if she has paralysis. In the early stages the aim is to help with breathing, coughing, eating and drinking; to turn the person to prevent pressure sores; and to position the limbs so as to prevent later complications such as spasticity (stiffness or tightness in the muscles and joints; see Glossary). Intermediate goals are to help the person sit, get out of bed, stand up, balance and walk alone. These activities are broken down into smaller tasks and the aim is to achieve some small goal in each session.

Trying to move when your muscle control is impaired and your sense of balance is poor can be a frightening experience. A physiotherapist can give practical help and encouragement to overcome this fear, which, if not tackled, can cause spasticity later. A physiotherapist will explain the causes of your relative's disabilities to you, and work with you to teach her rehabilitation techniques. Your relative will make most progress if you can work with her and the physiotherapist as a team, and encourage her to continue the exercises and techniques at home.

The occupational therapist

The role of the occupational therapist (OT) varies from place to place, but broadly it is to make the ordinary tasks of everyday living easier. An OT can help someone relearn day-to-day activities such as eating, dressing or getting in and out of the bath; make a home visit before discharge from hospital to assess the needs for, and recommend, aids and adaptations; give advice or teach your relative how to use them; and help find solutions to particular disabilities. An OT may give your relative advice about the best way to use muscles to promote recovery and prevent bad habits that could restrict movement later on.

He or she may be able to advise on claiming financial benefits and getting other support services, and can help someone wanting to return to work by showing how to reorganise work tasks to overcome disability.

The speech and language therapist

The speech and language therapist can identify problems with understanding, speaking, writing and reading, and diagnose the cause of these difficulties. Your relative should see a speech therapist as soon as possible if she has communication difficulties, especially if they are associated with swallowing problems. The speech therapist can diagnose the cause of swallowing difficulties, and help prevent complications such as dehydration, nutritional disorders and food or saliva entering the lungs.

Other therapists need to know the speech therapist's diagnosis, or they may try to communicate with the person in ways that are inappropriate. This can prevent accurate diagnosis of other problems. Communication difficulties can make a person seem stubborn and uncooperative. Unless you know how your relative's communication abilities have been affected, and what ways of communicating remain open to her, you and other people involved in her care may misunderstand the reasons for her behaviour.

Hospital nurses

Hospital nurses provide day-to-day care and advice. The ward nurse is a vital member of the stroke team, providing continuity of care and doing much of the rehabilitation. The nurse with overall responsibility for running the ward is the **sister** or **charge nurse** or **ward manager**. A **specialist nurse** provides advice on particular problems – for example, diabetes or incontinence – and may work with people in hospital and at home. A **hospital liaison nurse** is based in hospital but continues to give support when the patient returns home.

Psychiatric support team

People who have had a stroke and their carers often need support for the psychological effects of the illness. Emotional disturbance, anxiety, depression and mood disturbance are common after stroke. Carers also experience stress and depression. A **psychiatrist**, **psychologist** or **community psychiatric nurse** can help with these problems.

District nurse

District (community) nurses provide nursing support for people living at home in the community. They can help nurse your relative and show you how to do it, provide immediate aids such as a commode, hoist and walking stick, help rearrange the house to make caring for your relative easier, and show you how to handle and move your relative so as not to cause injury to her or yourself. A district nurse can also put you in touch with other agencies such as Meals on Wheels, stroke clubs or the social worker and give you practical advice and emotional support. The Patient's Charter says that in urgent cases you can expect a visit from someone in the district nurse team within four hours in the daytime.

Health visitor

Most health visitors work with families who have young children but some specialise in providing advice and support for older people living at home. They give advice about local services and benefits. Their main role is in health promotion and illness prevention.

Social worker

A social worker will assess your relative's needs for community care services (see p 54 for more information) and may help to arrange services such as Meals on Wheels, respite relief, day care, a home care assistant (home help), or aids and adaptations to help overcome disabilities. If your relative is returning home from hospital, a **hospital social worker** may provide a link between the hospital and the social services. The social worker will also advise on any benefits that your relative may be entitled to.

Getting the support that you need

According to the Patient's Charter, people have the right to receive health care on the basis of their clinical need. After a stroke, it is reasonable for your relative to expect an accurate diagnosis, and therapy to help recovery. The GP is the 'gatekeeper' to this care:

many GPs are excellent at opening doors, but others have to be persuaded. Don't hesitate to ask for what you need.

Keep yourself well informed

If your relative is in hospital, you need to know the extent of the stroke, the prospects of recovery and what progress your relative is making. You can ask to see the consultant if you feel you are not getting enough information. Make a list of questions or worries that you want to raise before meetings with any professionals; it's easy to forget what you wanted to ask.

Find out and plan for the likely discharge date

The ward sister or nursing manager should tell you when discharge is likely, explain what planning is needed, and may tell you about support services in the community. See page 50 for more information about planning for discharge from hospital.

Keep the GP well informed

Tell the GP about treatment your relative has received and let him or her know if you think additional help is needed. Managing care for someone who has had a stroke is a complicated task involving many different therapies and agencies. If your relative is unhappy with her GP, she has the right to change doctor. (If you want to make a formal complaint, see page 98 for information.)

Find out about other sources of information and support

Helpful books and leaflets on stroke are listed on the end of each chapter. The Stroke Association provides information, advice and support for people with stroke and carers, and produces a range of information leaflets. They and other organisations offering information, advice or support are listed in the Useful Addresses section. Also find out as much as you can about local sources of help. See pages 82 and 92 for suggestions.

Your best guarantee of obtaining the services that your relative needs is to arm yourself with information. Don't feel that you should simply accept the services offered. In some areas these will be excellent, but in other areas, if you don't ask, and keep on asking, your relative may miss out. If you know what you want and ask for it, you are more likely to get what your relative needs. If you don't get what is needed, the services will improve only if you and other carers tell them what would really help.

For more *i*nformation

ⓘ Stroke Association publications:

Leaflet S2 *Learning to speak again*

Booklet S7 *Stroke – a handbook for the patient's family*

Booklet S9 *Psychological effects of stroke*

Leaflet S14 *How occupational therapy helps stroke patients*

Leaflet S21 *Physiotherapy and strokes*

5 Planning for discharge from hospital

When someone who has had a stroke comes home from hospital is often a time of difficulty and stress. Good communication and planning can help to reduce the stress, but even with the best planning there are great adjustments to be made. For the person who has had the stroke it is a time of coming to terms with it and any disabilities it has left him with. He is no longer surrounded by skilled professionals and must start to rely on his own resources. For the carer it is the beginning of the demands of care and a time of major changes in her life.

This chapter helps you to plan for your relative's discharge from hospital. It gives you advice on what you need to know, the arrangements you need to make and the likely sources of help.

In case your relative is going to need continuing medical and nursing care, this chapter explains the hospital's responsibilities. It also gives information about patients' rights if the hospital wishes to discharge someone before they seem ready.

Patsy

'In the first few months when Leroy could do nothing I needed all the help I could get.'

'If I hadn't asked, I wouldn't have known when Leroy was coming out.

'One of the nurses gave me the address and telephone number of the Stroke Association regional office. They put me in touch with Sheila, who has been a great help. Sheila's been through it all herself and knows exactly where to go locally. In the first few months when Leroy could do nothing, I needed all the help I could get. Although I have retired, I had lots of other jobs outside the house with church and so on, and I also look after my granddaughter. Sometimes it seemed it was just work, work, work.'

Staying in control

When your relative leaves hospital can be very stressful if you are not ready for it. Before discharge, think about what your relative needs and what you need.

Start with your relative's needs; think of his:

- medical needs
- care needs
- social needs

Then look at your needs as a carer:

- how much time and work is caring likely to take?
- what are you prepared to take on?
- what help can you get?

The needs of the carer are dealt with in more detail in Chapter 6.

Your rights as patient and as carer

The Patient's Charter sets out your rights and the standards of service you can expect to receive from the NHS. The Government has also published guidelines on hospital discharge. The Patient's Charter says about leaving hospital:

'Before you are discharged from hospital, you can expect a decision to be made about how to meet any needs you may continue to have. Your hospital will agree arrangements with agencies such as community nursing services and local authority social services departments. You and, if you agree, your carers will be involved in making these decisions and will be kept up to date with information at all stages.'

When your relative returns home, the Patient's Charter says that:

'You can expect to receive a visit from someone in the district nurse team or the mental health nurse:

within 4 hours (in the daytime), if you have been referred to them as an urgent patient;

within 2 working days, if you have been referred to them as a non-urgent patient and you have not asked them to see you on any particular day; and

by appointment on the day you asked for, if you give the district nursing services more than 48 hours' notice.'

Government guidelines require hospitals to have a discharge procedure, to appoint one staff member to check that the procedure has been fully carried out and to make sure that all care arrangements are in place before a patient goes home. Patients and their carers or relatives have a right to be consulted and informed at every stage.

When will your relative be discharged?

The doctor in charge will decide when your relative is ready to leave hospital. If your relative is likely to have continuing care needs, the doctor should consult him and you before deciding the discharge date. When making a decision the doctor should take into account nonmedical matters affecting your relative's care, such as whether:

- your relative lives alone or with other people;
- there is anyone to care for your relative at home;
- the layout and arrangement of your relative's home are suitable for someone at his stage of recovery;
- the medical needs of your relative can be met at home;
- your relative is psychologically ready to return home;

- your relative's family is able to support him at home;
- the local authority support services are adequate.

The home environment and the level of care available at home are central concerns in the decision to discharge your relative. If you are the main carer, you should be involved in any discussions about your relative's discharge. You need to know how much and what type of care your relative requires. The hospital needs to know what care you can provide and what support will be available to you.

You have rights: use them

If you or your relative think that he is being discharged too early, speak to the ward sister or the consultant who makes the final decision about discharge. If you are seriously worried that you cannot provide the level of care that is being asked of you, don't feel you have to agree to it. The hospital has a duty to ensure that satisfactory arrangements have been made for your relative's safety when he returns home. Get advice from your local Community Health Council (called a Health Council in Scotland).

If your relative needs continuing care in a nursing home

Some people may need higher levels of continuing medical and nursing care after a stroke. Because many hospitals now discharge people earlier than they used to, the hospital may wish to discharge a patient to a nursing home.

Since 1 April 1996, Health Authorities have had to publish and operate policies, plans and eligibility criteria for a range of NHS continuing health care services, including rehabilitation, respite health care, specialist equipment and continuing inpatient care. Further details are contained in Age Concern England Factsheet 37 *Hospital discharge arrangements and NHS continuing health care services.*

If the hospital wishes to discharge your relative to a nursing home but he still has complex needs and requires a high level of care, find out what the health authority's policy says about who is eligible for NHS funding. If your relative is asked to pay for nursing home care, and you think he should be eligible for NHS funding, you may be able to ask for a review of the decision.

It may be helpful to talk to the hospital social worker. He or she works for social services but may be able to give advice about who is eligible for NHS funding. For fully independent advice, and for support if you wish to challenge a decision about NHS funding, contact your local Community Health Council (or Health Council in Scotland).

Deciding how to care for your relative

Before your relative is discharged from hospital you need to make a fairly sober decision about how to care for him in the future. Part of this decision concerns thinking about where would be best to care for him – will it be your home, his home, or a residential or nursing home? This is looked at in Chapter 6.

Try to talk to all the specialists involved about your relative's future care needs. Speak to the consultant and the different therapists and ask them for their assessment. With stroke it is impossible to say exactly how much someone will recover, but the hospital staff will be able to give you a general idea of your relative's likely recovery. Try to be as practical as possible in assessing your relative's needs (see Chapter 6).

How care and support are provided in the community

Community care assessment

Care provided at home by the health services and social services is now called community care. It is intended to provide a package of medical, nursing and social care tailored to individual needs that have been ascertained by a 'care assessment'. This assessment should identify the support that people need to enable them to continue to live in the community. Under the NHS and Community Care Act, local authorities are required to provide an assessment for anyone who appears to need community care services. Most local authorities have various levels of assessment. If your relative has considerable needs, there should be a full community care assessment. This is covered in more detail in Chapter 7 (see p 95).

An individual person may have care needs that require services from several different organisations, such as a hospital trust, the community nursing team, the home care team and providers of respite facilities. The provision of these services needs to be co-ordinated to make sure that nothing is overlooked. This is done by the care manager. This person could be a hospital social worker or someone from the local social services department (called the social work department in Scotland). When someone has many care needs, such as a person who has had a severe stroke, there may be a multi-disciplinary assessment. This will involve providers from different services and it is common practice in these circumstances to arrange a care management case conference. It will bring together all the different needs of your relative and provide a package of care designed to meet them. If you are the main carer, you may be invited to attend the conference.

If your relative is likely to need aids or adaptations to his home, an occupational therapist should carry out an assessment and make recommendations. The aids should be available before your relative leaves hospital, and any essential adaptations should also be completed. If they are not, a completion deadline should have been agreed with the local authority.

The hospital should tell your relative's GP when he is coming out, and provide medical details and requirements. A written discharge summary should be sent to your GP within 24 hours of discharge. The district nurse should have been notified and an appointment made for an early visit.

Ideally, hospital discharge procedures should ensure future care for your relative by smoothly transferring him to community care. If the system works efficiently, your relative's needs should be met.

If it doesn't, provision for your relative may fall short of what he requires. Even the best-run systems fail, so it is always worth checking that the necessary arrangements have been made. The following checklist will help you to do this. Find out who is the member of staff responsible for your relative's discharge and work through the checklist below.

Discharge checklist

Planned date of discharge _____

GP informed	Outpatient appointment made
Home visit requested	Medicines and aids received
Transport home arranged	

Clothes available	Food in house
House key available	Pension book returned
House warm	Valuables/money returned

Occupational therapist assessment completed; aids and adaptations installed/ordered	Physiotherapy arranged
	Occupational therapy arranged
District nurse requested	Speech and language therapy arranged
Health visitor requested	Continence adviser arranged

Social worker informed	Home help/Home care booked
Home care arranged	Day hospital/Rehabilitation arranged
Meals on Wheels booked	Respite care arranged

Sleeping arrangements assessed; aids and adaptations installed

Suitable seating arrangements assessed

Dressing arrangements assessed; aids and adaptations installed

Mobility assessed and aids provided

Access assessed; aids and adaptations installed

Cooking facilities assessed; aids and adaptations installed

Use of taps assessed; aids and adaptations installed

Heating equipment assessed; aids and adaptations installed

Suitable telephone installed

Washing facilities assessed; aids and adaptations installed

Facilities for bathing and showering assessed; aids and adaptations installed

Toilet facilities assessed; aids and adaptations installed

Voluntary sector organisations contacted:

❑ Age Concern ❑ Stroke Association ❑ Crossroads

Adapted, with permission, from *Going home from hospital* by Sheila White.

The importance of your relative's GP

Arrange for your relative to be seen by his GP soon after discharge to discuss his future health and care arrangements. If your relative has been given a 'discharge notification letter' for his GP, take it to the surgery. We have already seen (p 21) that the GP's active involvement in the management of your relative's care is essential to obtain access to health and care services. At the first visit, it is a good idea to arrange for your relative to see his GP after one week, after one month, after six months and then yearly. This enables the GP to monitor your relative's progress. If your relative is taking medication, he may need to see his GP more often.

What you need to know as a carer

Your own needs as a carer are covered in detail in Chapter 6. This section deals with what you need to know to help you care for your relative.

Nursing needs

If the person you care for is confined to bed and unable to turn himself, the nursing demands can be very heavy – turning him every two hours, day and night. The hospital therapists should explain your relative's problems and show you how to care for him. If your relative is paralysed, you need to know how to position his limbs, how to passively exercise his muscles and how to move him around. It is especially important never to pull him by his paralysed arm because it could damage his shoulder joint and lead to a frozen shoulder. The list below will help you to identify areas in which you may need help and instruction.

If your relative is confined to bed, how do you:

- move him to prevent pressure (bed) sores?
- turn him over?
- correctly place his limbs to prevent the development of spasticity?
- protect his paralysed limbs when turning him?
- help him to sit up?
- help him to move from bed to standing up?
- help him to move from bed to sitting in a chair?
- deal with incontinence?
- wash him?
- feed him if he has swallowing difficulties?
- prevent his becoming constipated?

If your relative can get out of bed himself, how do you:

- help him walk?
- help him eat?
- help him do exercises to prevent the development of spasticity?

Helping with rehabilitation

If your relative is paralysed or has speech difficulties, the therapists will have identified his problems and worked out exercises to help him. These exercises need to be continued at home to get the full benefit from them. It's best if you understand the reasons for the exercises because this will help you to do them properly. The therapists involved will give you this information. They will show you how to do the exercises, and explain what the problems are, how the exercises help and what they are trying to achieve.

Trial home visits

If you can, try to arrange a trial home visit before your relative is discharged from hospital. This will help you to spot unforeseen problems in the caring arrangements and give you a taste of what caring will be like. This will allow you to sort out any problems and to arrange more help if necessary.

Discharge from hospital is a difficult time even when carefully planned. In the Stroke Association survey *A Voice For Stroke*, 50 per cent of the people interviewed thought they had been discharged too early and only 36 per cent thought they had been given enough help. The more carefully you plan, the more manageable it will be. The Age Concern book *Going home from hospital* by Sheila White covers this important stage in greater detail than is possible here.

For more *i*nformation

i *Stroke! A self help manual for stroke sufferers and their relatives*, chapters 4 and 8, by Dr RM Youngson, published by David and Charles.

i *Going home from hospital* by Sheila White, published by Age Concern Books.

i Age Concern England Factsheet 37 *Hospital discharge arrangements and NHS continuing health care services*.

i Carers National Association Information Sheet 6 *Hospital Discharge*.

i The NHS Information Service, free advice on all aspects of healthcare: Freephone 0800 665544.

i *The Patient's Charter and You*, obtainable by dialling Freephone: 0800 66 55 44.

i Disablement Information Advice Line – DIAL (UK): 01302 310123.

i Stroke Association publications:

Leaflet S10 *On leaving hospital after a stroke*

Booklet S13 *Stroke and incontinence*

6 Providing care

In Britain over 90 per cent of caring is provided by family members, usually a partner or spouse. There are over 7 million unpaid carers, with 1.7 million heavily involved in hands-on care.

Caring can be very rewarding but can also be very demanding. Some carers feel that their life is changed beyond belief. They feel tired, stressed and angry, and sometimes isolated and despairing. But carers can also feel happy and confident.

The purpose of this chapter is to help you control what is happening in your lives. Caring for your relative is more likely to be rewarding if you recognise the problems, get sufficient support and acknowledge your own social and emotional needs.

Rosemary

'We all sat down and discussed what would be best.'

'Many people have no choice, but we did, and for us it seemed the right thing to do.

'Mum was very independent until she was 91. Then she had a series of minor strokes which left her feeling confused and weak on one side. I suggested Mum should come and stay on a temporary basis while we worked things out.

'My brother and his wife came over and we all sat down and discussed what would be best. Our children have left home so room wasn't a problem. My husband had retired and could give me a hand. My brother and his wife were still working full time, but they agreed to have her to stay from time to time to give us a break. They also helped to pay for any special aids or other things that Mum needs.

'We did our best to make Mum feel at home, by bringing things from her house and putting them in her room. We even brought her welsh dresser and put it downstairs.

'Mum did once go into a nursing home for a fortnight, while we had a holiday. But she wasn't happy there. It's not that they didn't look after her. Perhaps they did too much, because we noticed there were things she had been able to do for herself that she could no longer cope with.'

Are you able to care?

Most of us are able to respond to a short-term caring need by making do. However, this is no basis for long-term caring. If your relative does not go into hospital after her stroke, it is easy to slide from caring on this emergency basis to caring long term without thinking it through. If your relative goes into hospital, you usually have more time to reflect. Either way, it is important to consider fully your ability to provide longterm care and to look at the alternatives.

Long-term care – what you need to assess

Your relative's needs

You must have some idea of your relative's likely disabilities to assess realistically her long-term care needs. Talk to the doctor in charge of her case and to the different therapists to get their assessment.

61

Family involvement

Your relative must, of course, take as big a role as possible in coming to any decisions but remember to involve your other family members in discussing the options. You will then have a clear idea of what support you can expect from them.

Money matters

Caring for someone has big financial implications. You need to consider:

- loss of income for you and your relative;
- cost of caring and support services provided by the local authority or private sector;
- cost of aids and adaptations;
- cost of transport to hospital, outpatient clinics, day centres etc;
- your existing financial commitments;
- state benefits;
- pension rights;
- income from insurance policies;
- eligibility for grants for aids and adaptations;
- other income available to you and your relative.

Try to work out the financial implications by listing your income and taking away the likely costs. If you have difficulty in doing this, ask for help from your local Citizens Advice Bureau.

Pension rights

If your relative gets her pension from the post office, someone else can collect it for her by becoming her agent. Your relative can authorise this by writing the name of the person she wishes to be her agent on the back of the payment order and signing it. If she wants someone to collect her money regularly, that person can get an agency card from the local Benefits Agency office which allows them to do so.

If your relative is not capable of understanding what she is doing, the Benefits Agency can appoint you or somebody else to collect the money for her and spend it on her behalf.

Power of attorney If the power of attorney was signed after 1 January 1991 it will remain valid after the person giving it becomes mentally incapable. A solicitor will be needed to prepare the power of attorney. The application to the court for a **curator bonis** to be appointed is prepared by a solicitor, usually on behalf of a close relative of the person. Having a curator appointed is expensive and any professional will charge an annual administration fee. It is therefore not recommended for people with less than £15,000 of capital.

For more *i*nformation

ⓘ *Enduring Power of Attorney* and *Handbook for Receivers*, available free from the Court of Protection. Send a large sae to the address on page 127.

ⓘ *Managing Other People's Money*, published by Age Concern Books.

ⓘ *Dementia: Money and Legal Matters*, available free to carers from Alzheimer Scotland – Action on Dementia.

ⓘ Age Concern Factsheet 22 *Legal arrangements for managing financial affairs*, available from Age Concern Scotland.

How much help can you expect from social services?

What support you will be able to expect from social services depends on:

- your relative's needs;
- what services your local authority provides and what its charging policy is.

See pages 54 and 95.

Local voluntary organisations and support groups

Advice and information can often be obtained over the phone from voluntary organisations but support has to be local. Are there stroke or other support groups nearby? What respite services are available? What are the local opportunities for outings and holidays?

Support from neighbours, friends and the community

Is your local community supportive or can you expect little from your neighbours? Would a neighbour sit in with your relative while you went to the shops? Are you a member of a local church whose members might help? The amount of informal support can make a big difference, especially where voluntary agencies are thin on the ground.

Considering all the options

Before coming to any decisions, consider all the available options. The list below gives the broad options but you may have different possibilities locally: living at home with support; moving into sheltered housing; or moving into a residential or nursing home.

Living at home with support

In your joint home

If your relative lives with you and you are thinking of caring for her at home, consider the following:

- How mobile will she be?
- Will she be able to wash and dress herself and use the toilet without help?
- Will she need any special aids or equipment, or adaptations to the home?
- Will she be safe at home on her own, or will she need someone there all the time?
- What medicines will she need to take, what are they for, how should they be taken and when?
- Will she need any special diet; are there foods that she should or should not have?
- Will she need to attend an outpatient clinic or go into hospital for further tests or treatments; if so, how often?
- Can she get help with transport to hospital?
- What are the financial implications (see 'Money matters', above)?

Alone in her own home

If your relative lives alone and you care for her from a distance, the advantages are that she will:

- Retain her independence.
- Remain in familiar surroundings.
- Cope better in a familiar situation if her memory is affected.
- Keep in touch with friends and neighbours.
- Keep her support network intact.

The disadvantages are:

- The risk of further illness or injury – she may be willing to take this risk.
- Inadequate care.
- Loneliness, especially if she is housebound.
- Family too far away to visit.
- Adaptations being too expensive.

Moving home

Another possibility is one of you moving closer to the other. Again there are advantages and disadvantages. If you move, you may have to find a new job and you will lose contact with your own support networks. If your relative moves, she will lose the advantages of staying in her own home. If one of you moves into the other's home, there is the problem of loss of independence and the possibility of friction between you. If you move into your relative's home, you need to consider what would happen if she died or had to go into residential or nursing care. What right would you have to go on living in the property?

Sheltered housing

Sheltered housing is housing that includes some level of support for the occupants. The amount and type of support vary enormously with the scheme. Schemes are run by many different organisations – the local authorities, housing associations, charities and others. Most sheltered housing is rented but some can be bought. Look very carefully at the service costs if you consider buying; the additional charges may be as much as rent would be. Your local authority will tell you if your relative can get into a local authority scheme. If she cannot, ask them for a list of local housing associations that provide sheltered accommodation. Of the charitable organisations, Abbeyfield Houses are a popular choice. They are generally large houses with bedsits for up to about 10 older people, meals are provided and there is a resident housekeeper.

Moving into a care home

The possible advantages are:

- Safety.
- Full-time care.
- Trained staff.
- Good facilities.
- Possible companionship.
- No restrictions on your employment.
- Fewer demands on your time.

The possible disadvantages are:

- Uncertainty about the quality of care.
- Loss of independence.
- Unfamiliar surroundings.
- Loss of contact with family, friends and neighbours.
- Your relative may feel unwanted, unloved and unhappy.
- You and your family may feel guilty.
- The expense.
- The sale of your relative's home to meet the expense.

People on a low income or with savings below a certain amount (£16,000 in 1998) may get help with the cost of a care home.

If social services assess your relative as needing care in a home, they will make a financial assessment to decide how much she should pay towards the cost. If she has an income that is more than the cost of the care home, she will have to pay the full amount herself. If her income is less and her savings are below £16,000, social services will help with the costs.

If your relative needs to move into a care home permanently and she owns her own house or flat and lives alone, its value will be counted as part of her savings. This means she will have to pay the full cost of the care herself, until her savings have dropped to below £16,000. Most people arrange for their home to be sold. Your relative cannot be forced to sell her home but, if she chooses not to, the local authority has a legal right to put a charge on it. This means that, when the property is eventually sold, they have first claim on the proceeds to pay off the money she owes them.

Even if your relative is only going to move into a home temporarily, or is going to pay the full cost herself until her savings are reduced, it is still worth asking for a social services assessment. If social services agree that she needs to be in a care home, they may in some cases be able to negotiate a lower price on your relative's behalf than if she deals directly with the home herself.

Caring from a distance

If you are going to continue to live apart from your relative, there is still much you can do for her. If you live nearby, you can visit frequently and respond quickly to calls for help. You can help her sort out daily problems, provide meals and liaise with agencies such as the health service and the local authority social services.

If you live far away, you can still support her. Even if your relative has serious disabilities, do not assume she has to go into residential or nursing care. Community care may enable her to continue living in her own home: it all depends on the local services and the support of friends and neighbours. You can help by using the phone to make sure she gets the care services she needs and by contacting her regularly, daily if necessary, to check that she is all right.

Assessing your own needs as a carer

What does caring involve?

People who have never cared for a disabled person have little idea what caring entails. As a carer you need to recognise the reality of the task that you are taking on. If you do not, you are in danger of being swamped by it. Caring for a disabled person is difficult, but it need not be overwhelming if you can organise enough support.

The tiredness and bitterness you may feel as a result of caring are not caused by some deficiency in yourself: they are feelings shared by many carers. Research shows that:

- most full-time carers suffer from stress;
- the more hours spent caring each day, the greater the likelihood of ill health;
- nearly a half of carers feel under pressure;
- almost a quarter of carers feel at breaking point;
- two-thirds of carers have problems with budgeting.

Despite these experiences, the majority of carers feel they are coping well and are well supported.

Looking at your own needs

The key to successful caring is the amount of support you have. Financially secure carers who can take holidays when they wish and who feel well supported and valued also feel the most positive about caring. By arranging good support you will be looking after your own needs and those of your relative. Use the resource lists in this book to make sure you have sufficient support:

- to help you with physical tasks that are beyond you;
- to nurse and care for your relative;
- to have at least one day away from caring each week;
- to maintain a social life and outside interests;
- to have regular holidays;
- to give time to the rest of your family.

If you are thinking about giving up your job to care, consider the possibility of part-time work. A job provides more than just income: it provides self-esteem, social relationships, interests and a routine. Could you get by without these?

Respite care

'The single most important thing for me has been day care, it's what's kept me sane.'

'Dad didn't like going to the day centre but he went because he realised that, without the relief from caring, Mum couldn't cope.'

Respite care is care provided by others to give the main carer a break from caring. It may be only for an hour or long enough for a holiday abroad; it is available both at home and outside the home; it may be free or it may be charged for; it may be provided by the health service, local authority, voluntary organisations or the private sector. As many as 30 per cent of carers for older people who have had a stroke do not get a break from caring, although research carried out by the Carers National Association has shown that giving carers a break is the most effective way to help them carry on.

The cost of respite care will depend to some extent on where you live, what kind of care you and your relative need and which organisation arranges or provides it. It is a good idea to find out about the full range of respite care services that are available in your area before you make a decision. If respite care is arranged by the health service because your relative needs medical and/or nursing care, this should be free. If social services agree that you need respite care and arrange it on your behalf, they will make a financial assessment to decide how much you or your relative should contribute to the cost. (Charges vary from one social services department to another. Some services may be available free or at lower cost to people on low incomes. Some services are charged at the same rate to everyone.) Voluntary organisations that offer volunteer help may provide a free or low-cost service. Private organisations charge for their services. If social services arrange respite care with a voluntary or private organisation on your behalf, you may find the costs are different from those you would pay if you dealt with these organisations direct.

A regular break from caring is essential to prevent the burden of caring overwhelming you; many doctors recommend that you have at least one day a week away from your relative. Evidence shows that it is those caring for someone more than eight hours a day who find it most difficult to take a break when they want, yet it is these people who need it most. If your relative requires a high level of care, it is important both for you and your relative that you arrange adequate relief for yourself. If you do not, the likelihood is that you will become depressed and the quality of the care you can provide will decline.

Where to get respite care

Care for a few hours

Family, neighbours and friends.

Social services home care service – available seven days a week, covering such things as cleaning, laundry, making meals, shopping, collecting medicines, personal care, social skills support.

Voluntary sector respite services – provided by several voluntary organisations. Ask your local authority social services department for lists of organisations in your area or contact your local Voluntary Action/Council for Voluntary Service (CVS).

Crossroads Care – regular or occasional breaks for a few hours each week.

Small local schemes run by local churches and others – provide sitting, shopping, gardening, dog-walking services etc; contact them through your local Voluntary Action office or social services department.

Day care

Day centres run by social services provide a range of activities plus a midday meal for a small charge; contact your social services department to see if your relative is eligible.

Day hospitals – provided by the health service, accessed through your relative's GP or hospital doctor. They give help with medication, physiotherapy, occupational therapy, diagnosing health problems and nursing care.

Age Concern and other voluntary sector day centres; get information from your local social services department.

Private sector – care both at home and at day centres; get information from your local social services department.

Longer term respite – for days or weeks

Hospital respite care – periods of one or two weeks can be arranged on a regular basis. Make enquiries through your GP or hospital doctor; the final decision is made by a consultant.

Residential or nursing home respite care – means-tested for those who enter residential care on social services assessment system; the local health authority may pay for nursing home care. Contact social services for a list of approved homes.

Be flexible

The more flexible you are, the easier it is to find solutions. Even if your relative is severely disabled by stroke, it may be better to arrange care for her that is shared with others rather than to take it on alone. A combination of day care, home care services, support from family and neighbours, voluntary organisation care and private sector care may allow you to carry on working, at least part-time.

The key to flexibility is information. The main sources of information for carers are friends, charities and social services. Try to make use of all sources of information – GPs, hospitals, telephone helplines, public libraries, newspapers and the radio. The more you know, the easier it is to find a solution.

Making a decision

When facing difficult problems it is easy to become frozen in indecision. The different possibilities go round and round in your head and events drift along, dragging you with them.

Many people find that using a simple decision-making technique helps to prevent this from happening and keeps them in control of their own lives. The stages of the technique are quite simple:

1 List the problems.
2 Sort them into their order of importance.
3 Starting with the most important problem, list all the different solutions to the problem you can think of.
4 Choose the solution that you think will work best.
5 Carry out the solution.
6 Go on to the next problem.

Sometimes just listing the problems helps you to see more clearly where to start. Slicing a big problem into smaller manageable sized slices is often called 'the salami technique'.

Caring for yourself

Starting to care for someone who has had a stroke is often a traumatic experience. It brings anxiety, major changes in roles and relationships and permanent changes in your life-style. These changes are stressful. The risk of depression for the carer is real – about a third of carers experience depression and more than half feel that their health has suffered. Try to think about the steps you can take to prevent this happening to you.

■ Recognise how your relative's stroke affects your emotions. Many people go through a grieving stage for their lost life. Talk to your friends and relatives about it. If this doesn't help, speak to the community psychiatric nurse or your GP.
■ Organise others to support you in your daily caring routine. Accept help offered by friends and neighbours. Get help early.
■ Take regular time off from caring.
■ Take regular holidays.

- Do not let yourself become socially isolated. Your social life may change – you have new interests and responsibilities – but make sure you have one.
- Join a stroke club, carers group or support group. Other people who understand what you and your relative are going through can make a big difference.
- Encourage your relative to be as independent as possible right from the start, for both your sakes.

For more *i*nformation

i *Disabled in Britain: Behind closed doors – the carers' experience*, published by Scope (formerly The Spastics Society).

i *Finding and paying for residential and nursing home care* by Marina Lewycka, published by Age Concern Books.

i *The Carer's Handbook: What to do and who to turn to* by Marina Lewycka, published by Age Concern Books.

i *A Voice for Stroke*, published by the Stroke Association.

i Stroke Association publications:

Booklet S7 Stroke: *A handbook for the patient's family*

Booklet S9 *Psychological effects of stroke: a guide for the carer*

Leaflet S10 *On leaving hospital after a stroke*

i Age Concern Factsheet 10 *Local authority charging procedures for residential and nursing home care* explains social services systems for charging in more detail.

i Age Concern Factsheet 6 *Finding help at home.*

i Age Concern Factsheet 29 *Finding residential and nursing home accommodation.*

Caring for your relative at home

Many people go through a period of feeling dejected after returning home from hospital. As they face up to living with their new disabilities, the contrast between life before and life after stroke is at its starkest, but expert help is no longer on hand to reassure them. Your relative may suddenly feel very much on his own as he realises that living with stroke is now the everyday reality.

For the carer, too, there are the practical tasks to be done; the frustration of dealing with bureaucracies and caring agencies that appear not to care; the distress at seeing the rate of recovery start to slow down; big adjustments to make in day-to-day living; and, above all, the physical demands of caring.

This chapter discusses the needs and difficulties you may face caring for someone at home, and suggests where to go for help.

Jane

'Joining the stroke club was a great help: meeting other people, swapping experiences, listening and talking.'

'My father-in-law sat in a chair for thirty years. I was determined that it was not going to happen to Fred.

'At first I was in a state of shock; nobody ever explained what happened, I had no back-up at all and I found it very hard. Fred thought everyone was against him, even me, he used to get very tearful. It was only when a friend who was a care assistant said we needed help that we got anything: then we got Meals on Wheels and a home help and Fred started going to the day centre. Joining the stroke club was a great help: meeting other people, swapping experiences, listening and talking. It helps so much, especially when you meet other people who are worse off than you, and you can help them.

'Stroke is such a terrific thing that, however things were before, they are going to be different afterwards, but we still fight it, we still won't give in. We go on holidays three times a year and Fred drives the camper. We've had to stop joining things – there are only so many societies that you can manage.'

Emotional and psychological aspects of stroke

The reality of stroke

You and your relative will need time to come to terms with the effects of the stroke. A severe stroke means real losses in ability, independence and hopes for the future, and changes in family and social relationships. A life change like this has emotional and psychological effects, and, although each person finds his or her own way of coping, reactions often follow a common pattern. You may recognise some of these in yourself, or in the person you care for:

Shock and disbelief – a feeling that what is happening is not real, that you will wake up and all will be well again.

Denial – a refusal to accept the consequences of what has happened. This can last for days or months. It protects us from being overwhelmed by the change in our lives, but we can get stuck in denial and never come to terms with our new circumstances.

Anger – at oneself and at others: at doctors for not doing enough, at carers for not caring, at the ill person for having a stroke in the first place or not appreciating what is done for him.

Grief – for what has been lost; looking back to how life was before the stroke. Grieving can be a long-term process, involving other feelings (anxiety, anger, guilt) at different stages.

Anxiety – fear of walking unaided or being alone, fear of death or another stroke, fear that the carer may die or become incapacitated, fear of meeting other people or of going out. The carer may fear that the person cared for will die or have another stroke.

Guilt – about how the stroke has caused such disruption to everyone's lives, about being dependent, about no longer being able to work, about not being able to contribute as before. Carers may worry that they somehow caused the stroke, or feel guilty about the difficult, negative feelings they have towards their relative. That this guilt is irrational and unfounded does not make it any less powerful and destructive.

Acceptance and adjustment – with time, there is a gradual coming to terms with and adjusting to the new situation. This is healthy so long as the adjustment is positive, seeking to make the best of things rather than resignation or despair.

These psychological changes are often associated with physical effects, too:

- a great need to cry;
- tiredness, difficulty in getting to sleep, disturbed sleep, restlessness or sleeping too long;
- loss of appetite, indigestion, or an upset stomach, diarrhoea or constipation;
- palpitations (unusual heart beat);
- weight loss;
- the carer experiencing symptoms that mimic the effects of stroke.

The physical effects are upsetting but generally ease with time. Nevertheless, if powerful feelings or physical symptoms are affecting your own or your relative's ability to cope, ask your GP for help.

Problems with day-to-day activities

The abilities to eat, talk, walk, dress, wash and use the toilet without assistance are central to our sense of independence and adulthood. Encourage your relative to recover these abilities. If there are specific problems, get advice early on how to overcome them.

Because these abilities are so vital to self-esteem, your relative is likely to invest a lot of energy in trying to achieve them. Even small failures may trigger a disproportionate emotional outburst. If this happens, try not to criticise. Remember that emotional instability is one of the effects of stroke, especially in the early months. Ignore abuse and try to talk calmly through what went wrong. Help your relative to be specific about the problem. Then look for a practical solution. For example, 'I feel completely useless and a waste of space' could be expressing understandable anger and frustration at the difficulty of handling food that is not cut up small enough. Understanding what triggers strong emotions can help to avoid problems in future.

See pages 43–49 and the chart on pages 92–95 for information about professionals and services that can help your relative regain independence.

Psychological problems

Anxiety

Anxiety can be a serious problem if it prevents your relative doing what he could otherwise do. For example, someone who is quite happy to walk unaided around the home may panic at the idea of going outside. Worry about falling is a real fear, for which there are practical solutions. But anxiety is often a sign of some underlying, unspoken fear, which may be unfounded: 'If I walk too much I will provoke another stroke'. If the unfounded fear is not tackled it can grow, and anxiety about going outside may become a fear of walking at all.

What you can do to help

- Keep a diary for about a week to identify what situations your relative seems to avoid unnecessarily.
- Find out what it is about the situations that make your relative anxious.
- Get your relative to put anxiety-provoking thoughts into words.
- Find a solution to any real practical problems.
- Work through the anxiety-provoking thoughts by asking:
  - what evidence is there to support this belief?
  - is there any other explanation?
  - what would help cope with the situation?
- Build up confidence by gradually exposing your relative to the feared situation:
  - break the task into small steps, each one building on the previous step and encouraging greater independence;
  - don't move on to the next stage until your relative can confidently do what is required at this stage;
  - if there are setbacks don't give up: work out why and go back to a stage where your relative feels confident;
  - build in rewards along the way – but keep in mind that the real reward is overcoming the fear.

Anxiety can cause tension, headache and tiredness. Learning how to relax properly can help. Most bookshops and libraries have books on different kinds of techniques for learning relaxation. Or ask your GP, physiotherapist, occupational therapist or community psychiatric nurse.

If anxiety is a serious problem, your relative needs to discuss it with a doctor or community psychiatric nurse.

Depression

'The depression is almost worse than the immobility.'

> 'Neither of us could shake off the depression until we spoke to the community psychiatric nurse; counselling made all the difference.'

Feelings of loneliness, emptiness or despair are natural and not uncommon in the early days, but there is a risk of longer-term depression, which may need to be treated. Depression distorts the way we see the world, so a depressed person tends to over-generalise from one thing to the whole of life – 'If I can't do this, I can't do anything'. It can make the person feel guilty – 'I've not only ruined my life, I've ruined my family's as well' – and it drastically undermines self-esteem.

These thoughts, though unfounded, tend to further undermine well-being and deepen the depression. Somehow the downward spiral must be broken. Sometimes it helps to look at depressing thoughts objectively, to identify specific problems and work out possible solutions. If there is not a real problem, it can help to make a list of all the arguments which show that the problem is imaginary, and refer to them whenever the depressing thoughts come back.

If you or your relative gets stuck in depression for more than two weeks, you need help. Speak to your GP or community psychiatric nurse. Do it sooner rather than later; the earlier you get help, the more effective it is. Your GP may refer you to a psychiatrist or clinical psychologist who will help you to define your problems and give you treatment to overcome them.

The doctor may prescribe antidepressant drugs which lift depression by altering mood. These often take up to ten days to start working, and need monitoring because they may have unpleasant side effects, especially in older people. They may also be incompatible with other medication. The side effects often wear off after a few weeks as the body adjusts to the drug, or the doctor may try to avoid side effects by starting with small doses and gradually building up to an effective dose. Besides improving mood, antidepressants also help in other ways: appetite increases, sleep improves and the person has more energy. These all help to overcome the depression.

Tranquillisers are best avoided in the treatment of depression because they dull responses, do not alter mood, can cause loss of balance and can be addictive.

There is evidence that, although depression affects about one in three stroke patients and a similar number of carers, GPs often overlook it. If your GP is not able to help, there may be a hospital or community psychiatric team who can. In some areas you can contact the team direct, though it is better not to bypass the GP.

Isolation

Isolation can be a real problem. Loss of mobility and/or difficulty in talking can make it hard to keep in touch with people. The demands of caring also limit the carer's social life. The carer and the person cared for may have to give up work, and both may have to give up other activities that they enjoy.

> 'People are very kind and invite us round for meals and a get-together, but Eddie doesn't like to go because he's embarrassed that he needs help with eating – I don't know why he's bothered, it doesn't really matter, everyone realises that he has difficulties, they want him there for his company and what he has to say, not the way he eats.'

What you can do to help

Get help with practical difficulties A speech and language therapist can help with communication difficulties. Dial-a-Ride, social services and local voluntary organisations may help with transport. Motability and the Benefits Agency can give advice about getting a specially adapted car. (See page 120 for more about driving after a stroke.)

Talk to friends about your relative's disability Your relative may withdraw from seeing people out of embarrassment, or out of concern that friends will feel embarrassed by his disabilities. Explain to them, if necessary, where to sit and how to say things to make it easier for your relative.

Reintroduce your relative to social situations gradually Start by bringing an old friend to the house, then several, then go out to meet someone in their house, then go to a pub or a cafe and so on.

Old friends can help if your relative's recent memory has been affected. They can talk about things that happened years ago, which your relative will find easier to recall. They can help to place new events in this familiar landscape, and this will help your relative to understand and remember them.

Think about joining your local Stroke Club Other people in the club have been through and understand the difficulties that you and your relative face; they can offer practical advice and emotional support. Club events and trips are a good way of building up confidence in dealing with social situations. In overcoming isolation, nothing succeeds like success.

Caring for someone whose character has changed

It is often said that stroke changes people's personalities. This idea is distressing, but it is usually not the case. What happens is that stroke changes *an aspect* of somebody's character. Understanding this opens up the possibility of doing something about it.

A stroke often leads to depression, for example, which can make a person miserable. The stroke then seems to have changed a previously happy personality into a miserable one. But this is not the real problem. The problem is the depression, which *can* be treated. Other psychological changes such as aggressiveness, abusiveness and avoiding social contact can also be treated. Don't simply accept 'personality' problems. Ask your relative's GP for a referral to a psychiatrist, clinical psychologist or psycho-geriatrician, who can do something about them.

Common psychological changes

Be aware that psychological changes are as much the effects of stroke as a paralysed arm or leg. Reassure your relative that they are not signs of madness or dementia, and that they *can* be helped. These are some of the common ones:

- Tiredness, especially when reading, talking or doing mental work.
- Loss of concentration.
- Loss of initiative.
- Poor short-term memory (this memory loss is common and often does not improve).
- Irritability, especially in people who have had a right hemisphere stroke.
- Inability to handle stressful situations.
- Fear and anxiety – about further strokes, falling, permanent disability or insufficient money.
- Anger – aggressive outbursts towards the carer and others.
- Frustration, especially if your relative's ability to communicate has been damaged.
- Uncontrolled swearing, which will probably distress your relative as much as you.
- Weepiness or excessive laughter – you can help your relative get over these by changing to a topic of conversation that is not emotionally charged.
- Emotional outbursts combining frustration, anger and depression when your relative finds he can't do something that he could previously do with ease. It is important not to ask your relative to do things beyond his capabilities.

(Adapted from *Practical Management of Stroke* by Graham P. Mulley, Chapman and Hall, 1988. Not currently in print but available in libraries.)

The effect of stroke on the whole family

Stroke affects the whole family. Other family members, as well as the carer, have to come to terms with the stroke and its implications, face decisions about the practical tasks of caring and support, and adjust to new roles. When there are young children in the family there are additional emotional and practical concerns. In the early days, family members may seek reassurance from each other about the seriousness of the stroke and its likely outcome. People often need to go over the same ground again and again. This helps us understand and adapt to the situation, and face up to future possibilities.

Families with young children

Families whose children are still dependent on their parents face a range of problems if one of the parents has a stroke. There are practical problems caused by the loss of income and the new caring responsibilities, and there are emotional and psychological problems as the family adjusts to the new situation.

The unaffected partner often has to take on the bulk of the responsibility for caring for the children and to cope with tasks such as housework or the family finances previously handled by the spouse. If the carer is employed, a sensible solution to the additional responsibilities often appears to be to stop working to allow extra time for caring. This decision should be thought through very carefully, as it probably means less income and less social contact for the carer. Ultimately, it might reduce the carer's ability to cope rather than improving it.

The parent who has had the stroke will have to develop a new relationship with his children. This can be a difficult adjustment if he has significant communication or physical disabilities. He may no longer be able to care for his children and the children may no longer accept him in a parental role. It is important for his self-esteem that he is not placed in situations with the children that he cannot handle. The occupational therapist can give advice on how to lift children and care for them with one hand and ParentAbility can give advice and support.

The psychological and emotional strains in these circumstances are substantial and need to be recognised so that help is sought when it is needed. The parent who has had the stroke often experiences depression, intense guilt, anger and frustration at not being able to carry out his role and support the family in the old way. The carer often shares similar emotions plus resentment at the additional demands placed on her. A common response to these emotions is to feel ashamed of them and to try to suppress them but this will probably only make them worse. They need to be acknowledged as a normal response to a very difficult situation and help sought in coming to terms with them.

Practical, emotional and psychological support are essential in this situation. Advice on where to get this support is given in this chapter and throughout the book. The Stroke Association produce a very helpful booklet, S20 *Stroke in younger adults*, which contains excellent advice and lists of support organisations.

Planning for the future

Try to involve the whole family in making decisions; remember to include relatives outside the immediate family. If you are the main carer, it is important to be able to say to other members of the family exactly what support you need. Most people have no idea of what caring for another adult is like. It is only by explaining your needs to them and, if possible, involving them in the practical caring that they will begin to understand what you have to deal with. Involving everyone can also help prevent future misunderstanding and argument. The other thing to recognise is that situations change. Plans may need to be altered later, and it helps if everyone involved is prepared to be flexible.

Adapting to nursing and caring roles

Adapting to new nursing and caring roles isn't easy. We all tend to live our lives to the full. Caring for someone who is heavily dependent inevitably means a big shift in priorities, for all the family.

Other roles

It helps to encourage your relative to take on responsibilities within the family *right from the start*. He may no longer be able to fulfil his former role, which can damage his self-esteem. Other family members may have to take over parts of this role, which can cause resentment. Responsibility that he *can* cope with will help to boost your relative's self-confidence and maintain the respect of other family members.

Encouraging independence

Having adopted a caring role, people sometimes find it difficult to encourage independence in their relative. But it is essential to do so. Re-achieving independence takes considerable effort. Tasks that were once done without thought now prove unbearably difficult, and you are more than likely to bear the brunt of the resulting anger and frustration. You may be accused of not caring or not understanding the difficulties. If you take these feelings at face value, they can make *you* feel angry, resentful and bitter. Try to see them for what they are – a not unreasonable response to a seemingly impossible situation. Someone with a stroke needs a lot of encouragement and motivation. Try not to be critical, but don't keep your own feelings bottled up. You need to find someone who understands – perhaps other family members, friends, a counsellor or a sympathetic health professional – whom you can talk to frankly about how you're feeling.

It may help to set down firm limits about what you will and will not do and how often, in order to motivate your relative and stretch his abilities. Sometimes a person who has had a stroke asks for a very great deal of time and attention, so you can't get any time for other tasks, or for yourself. You may be able to talk things through and explain you have needs too, and come to an agreement. But if you can't do this, explain clearly what you are and are not prepared to do and stick to it. Be persistent. It is easier in the short term to do things *for* someone, but real compassion lies in helping your relative to become as independent as possible.

Your feelings about caring

Caring is stressful. The points when you are likely to feel very stressed are:

- when the stroke happens;
- when your relative leaves hospital;
- when rehabilitation support ends.

No one can predict a stroke but, once it has happened, it helps if you can find out when the other events will be and plan to make the changes as smooth as possible. Above all, you need to organise support for yourself through these stages, from family, friends and neighbours, and from professionals.

It is common for carers to build up feelings of resentment against the person they care for. The first thing to recognise is that these feelings are absolutely normal. They are a natural response to a stressful situation and should not make you feel guilty. It can help to talk your feelings through with someone else, perhaps another family member, a friend or a sympathetic professional. If there is a stroke club in your area, it may help to talk to other members of the club who will understand exactly what you are going through. Just talking can help you get your feelings into perspective and help you to identify real problems.

Sometimes feelings can get out of hand. If you feel you cannot cope any longer, or are worried that you might neglect or even abuse your relative, you need to get help. Speak to your GP or community psychiatric nurse, and try to tell them honestly how you are feeling. They may be able to arrange a break from caring, or more practical help in the home, or perhaps counselling.

Carer and partner

Caring for a partner can put your role as a partner under stress. When someone else is heavily dependent on you, it's difficult to think of them as a full and active partner in the relationship.

Severe disability or loss of language can make carers feel that they have lost their former partner, and carers often go through a process of grieving for this loss. It may take anything between six months and two years to come to terms with these feelings, and to find new activities that you can enjoy with your partner.

A partner's disabilities impose restrictions on the carer, which can fuel feelings of resentment. The first thing to do is recognise these feelings. They are a normal response to stress, and nothing to feel guilty or ashamed about. Once you have acknowledged your feelings, you can start to do something about them.

Try to identify practical problems that contribute to negative feelings. For example, make a list of the activities that your partner's disabilities prevent you from doing. Put them in order of importance, and try the problem-solving technique outlined on page 74 to help find solutions.

If your relationship was already under strain before the stroke, the stress of caring is likely to make it worse. Sometimes counselling can help. Relate (see Useful Addresses) is an organisation that offers counselling and support for difficulties in relationships. The earlier you get help, the more effective it is likely to be.

Sex

Many couples stop having sex after a stroke, for all sorts of reasons. A common one is the belief that sex may precipitate another stroke. For most people, there is no evidence that it will, but someone with high blood pressure who has had a haemorrhage-type stroke should get advice from the doctor. It may be difficult to make love if a partner is paralysed, but experiment. Your partner may be able to lie on the weak side, leaving the active arm free. Certain drugs prescribed for blood pressure or blood circulation problems, depression, anxiety or sleeplessness can make it difficult to have an erection. Speak to your GP, who may try a different drug.

Making love is an essential part of many relationships, whatever the partners' ages. It is a way of expressing love for each other, helps to relieve stress and cements the relationship. If both you and your partner wish to continue sex after the stroke but there is a practical problem, it can almost certainly be overcome with the right advice. If only one partner wishes to continue a sexual relationship, it could become a source of tension if not resolved. It is well worth getting advice, sooner rather than later.

Sources of help

Ask your GP, who may be able to help you directly or refer you to an advisory agency or someone in the psychiatric support team. There are many books on sex, available in bookshops and libraries. Four in particular that may be helpful are listed below.

For more *i*nformation

🛈 *Enjoy Sex in the Middle Years* by Dr Christine Sandford, published by Macdonald Optima.

🛈 *The Joy of Sex* by Dr Alex Comfort, published by Quartet.

🛈 *Living, Loving and Ageing* by Wendy Greengross and Sally Greengross, published by Age Concern Books.

🛈 *Vitality and Virility* by Neil Davidson, published by Age Concern Books.

🛈 The Stroke Association Leaflet S16 *Sex after stroke illness.*

🛈 The Association to Aid the Sexual and Personal Relationships of the Disabled (SPOD). See Useful Addresses.

Seeking and accepting help

Many people feel reluctant to ask for help, but caring for someone with disabilities caused by stroke is physically and mentally draining, whatever your age. Three-quarters of carers for stroke sufferers are over 60 themselves, and are likely to need help with the demands of caring. If you don't get enough help and support, the stress could make you ill yourself.

Work out what you need most and think about all the different sources of help that you could draw on: family, friends, neighbours, church, trades union, voluntary organisations, local support and self-help groups, the health service, your local authority, especially the social services department, and the Benefits Agency (social security). See also the chart on pages 92–95. If you can arm yourself with information and start organising your own support early, coping in the long term will be easier.

Long-term care in Britain depends heavily on unpaid care. According to the British Medical Association, unpaid carers in Britain provide up to £39 billion worth of care. Given their enormous contribution to society, carers have every right to expect some help from health and social services. But, because of limited resources, both central and local government have to ration how much help is provided. If you have difficulty getting what you need, it is not necessarily because your needs are unreasonable. You may need to be persistent. Ask, and keep on asking.

If your relative has needs which you believe *should* be met by social services, and you think you may have been unfairly treated, you can ask to speak to the officer who deals with complaints to get advice or to find out how to make a formal complaint (see pp 98–99). If your own or your relative's needs or circumstances change, you are entitled to ask social services for a reassessment of needs (see p 100 for more information).

Dealing with officials

Always find out the name of the person you are speaking to and write it down in a notebook you keep for this purpose.

- Write down any promises the person makes and the date the promise was made.
- Follow up any promises that fail to materialise. Speak to the person who made the promise, or, if this doesn't help, speak to a superior.
- Because of the limited resources, you may find it difficult to get help unless there is a crisis, or you are at breaking point. It is sometimes necessary to show the person involved that you may no longer be able to cope if you don't get help.

Practical help with caring

If your relative is not admitted to hospital

The doctor who first sees your relative will assess whether he should be admitted to hospital. If this is not necessary, the GP will be the key person in managing his care. The GP can refer your relative to other professionals, and arrange access to other services that he needs. See page 43 for more information about health services for someone who has had a stroke.

The local authority social services department may be able to arrange help such as Meals on Wheels, help with housework or shopping, a break from caring, or equipment for daily living. Contact social services through your relative's GP or the occupational therapist (see p 45), or phone the social services office for your area (in the phone book under the name of your local council) and ask the duty officer for information.

Where to get help

Services vary widely from place to place. The checklist below gives you an idea of what help *may* be available, and whom to contact for more information.

Checklist of support services at home

Help with housework, shopping, cleaning	*Social services, voluntary organisation or private agency*
Help with getting up, getting washed and dressed, going to the toilet, eating, getting undressed, going to bed	*Social services or voluntary care attendant scheme (eg Crossroads) or private agency (eg Care Alternatives)*
Help with incontinence or incontinence supplies (pads, pants, bedding)	*District nurse or continence adviser (ask the GP)*

Help with nursing, bathing, toileting, lifting	*District nurse (ask the GP) or private nursing agency*
Laundry service	*Social services (many areas no longer offer this service) (look in the* Yellow Pages)
Meals on wheels	*Social services, local community group, church or voluntary group*
Advice about most general health problems	*Your relative's GP who may refer him to someone else*
Nursing care at home, eg injections, changing dressings	*District nurse (ask the GP) or private nursing agency*
Advice about lifting or turning someone heavy	*District nurse or physiotherapist or occupational therapist(ask the GP)*
Advice on mobility and exercise	*Physiotherapist (ask the GP)*
Foot care, help with nail cutting	*NHS chiropodist (ask the GP or district nurse) or private chiropodist*
Advice on equipment to help with everyday living, eg washing, cooking, using the toilet	*Occupational therapist (social services department or hospital) or disabiled living centre (contact the Disabled Living Centres Council)*
Equipment for bedroom (rails, hoist, etc)	*District nurse or occupational therapist (social services)*
Mobility aids, eg wheelchair, walking sticks, walking frames	*GP, physiotherapist or hospital (ask the GP)*
Short-term hire of equipment	*British Red Cross (ask at the local branch), local Age Concern group, the WRVS or other organisations*

Adaptations to make your home more suitable for a disabled person	*Occupational therapist (social services department, housing or environmental health department), or voluntary organisation (eg Care and Repair)*
Help with transport	*Dial-a-ride or other voluntary organisation, social services or private taxi*
Transport to and from voluntary luncheon club, day centre, etc	*Social services or community group*
Transport to shops	*Community or voluntary group, Good Neighbour scheme (ask at social services). Some large stores run a bus service*
Advice about getting a specially adapted car	*Motability, Department of Social Security*
Orange parking badge	*Social services*
Disabled Person's Railcard	*Local (staffed) railway station*
Day centre, luncheon or social club	*Social services, voluntary organisation (eg local Age Concern) or community centre*
Holidays	*Social services or voluntary group (eg Carers National Association), Holiday Care Service*
Someone to sit with your relative while you go out for a few hours	*Social services, voluntary organisation (eg Crossroads) or private agency (eg Care Alternatives)*
Day care for your relative in a special centre; may include lunch, social activities, use of bathing facilities, chiropody, hairdressing, etc	*Social services, hospital or voluntary organisation (eg Age Concern, Help the Aged or Alzheimer's Disease Society)*

| Short-term care away from home, from a day to a fortnight. Could be in a hospital, residential or nursing home, or even with another family | *Social services, hospital, private or voluntary residential or nursing home* |

Adapted, with permission, from *The Carer's Handbook: What to do and who to turn to* by Marina Lewycka.

Contacting social services: community care assessment

The occupational therapist or a social worker from the community health team may arrange a community care assessment (see p 54), or your GP may arrange for a social worker to come to see you. If this doesn't happen but you think your relative needs support, contact social services direct and ask about an assessment.

If you are providing a substantial amount of care to your relative on a regular basis, under the Carers (Recognition and Services) Act 1995, which came into effect on 1 April 1996, you have the right to ask the local authority to also consider your needs when they are assessing the needs of your relative.

Make sure you give as much information as you can about your relative's needs at your first contact with social services. The duty officer who answers your first telephone call may make an initial assessment of your relative's needs and decide whether a fuller assessment is necessary. Because full assessments are expensive, they are done only if social services considers them essential. A serious stroke justifies a full assessment because your relative's needs are likely to be extensive and require support from a range of different services.

Make sure you explain:

■ The extent of your relative's disability and what this prevents him doing for himself. Be specific: can't get out of bed, can't use the toilet, can't feed himself, can't cook or prepare food, can't bath, can't walk.

■ What aids or equipment you think your relative needs. (Get advice from the occupational therapist if you can: see p 45.)

■ How the house needs to be adapted to help you care for your relative; for example, ramps for wheelchairs, a stair lift, a downstairs bathroom or widening of doorways. (Ask the occupational therapist for advice.)

■ How much care your relative needs: does he need someone with him every moment of the day and night, or does he just need someone to prepare his meals?

■ How much care you can provide: mention your age, any health problems you have, and other obligations such as a job or caring for someone else. Explain any practical difficulties, such as being unable to lift your relative. Think through caring for your relative in as much practical detail as you can – for example, you might have bouts of rheumatism or arthritis which prevent you doing things on some days that you could do easily on others – and list any problem areas.

■ What help your relative needs to get about outside the house.

■ What help your relative needs to participate in social and leisure activities.

This is a lot of information to prepare, and you may find it helpful to work through these points with a friend or another family member. Make a list of the details so that you can refer to it when you telephone the social services department, and use it at the care assessment meeting if this takes place.

You can ask for a reassessment if your relative's or your needs change. See page 100.

Financial assessment

Some community care services are free, some are charged at a flat rate for everyone and some are means-tested – whether and how much a person is charged depends on their ability to pay. The system for paying for care at home will depend on the local authority where the person lives. But there is a national means-testing system for residential and nursing home care, unless the health authority buys or funds the place in the home. (See Age Concern's Factsheet 10.) A person who has income or savings above a certain level will be asked to contribute towards the cost of means-tested services. This operates on a sliding scale: for example, if your relative has savings above £16,000 he would currently have to pay the full cost of a care home. If your relative goes into a nursing or residential home permanently and he owns his own home, in certain circumstances this too may be regarded as savings. See page 69 for more information.

It may distress your relative to know that his finances are to be assessed. It may help to explain what will happen and that a financial assessment is required by law. Point out that there may be advantages: he may not have to pay the full cost of services, and he may find that he is entitled to Social Security benefits.

Other sources of help

Voluntary organisations

Voluntary organisations can offer different kinds of practical help and support:

Age Concern – advice, information, publications and practical help for older people.

Carers National Association – support, advice, information and publications for carers.

Citizens Advice Bureau – advice and information about benefits, debts, housing and employment.

Crossroads Care – respite care.

DIAL UK– advice and information for disabled people and their carers.

Disabled Living Foundation and Disabled Living Centres – showrooms and advice on aids and equipment for disabled people.

RADAR – information about equipment, mobility, leisure, sport, etc for people with disabilities.

Stroke Association – advice, information, publications and practical support for people who have had a stroke and their families (in Scotland it is called Chest, Heart and Stroke, Scotland, and in Northern Ireland it is called the Northern Ireland Chest, Heart and Stroke Association).

For more information about these organisations and how to contact them, see the Useful Addresses section. Most organisations have local branches or groups. The Disabled Living Foundation can put you in touch with your nearest Disabled Living Centre.

Resources in your community

There are many other local organisations that provide advice and practical support, and some run self-help groups. Find out more from the social services department or your local Council for Voluntary Service/Voluntary Action/Rural Community Council, the local co-ordinating body for voluntary groups; you can get their telephone number from the Councils for Voluntary Service National Association enquiry line (0114 278 6636) or in Scotland from the Scottish Council for Voluntary Organisations (0131-556 3882).

Setting up a stroke club/support group

If there is no stroke club in your area, you could consider setting one up. The Stroke Association will help you to do this. Their free leaflet S4, *Starting a stroke club/stroke support group*, has advice on how to go about it.

If you cannot get the help you need

You may find that you cannot get the help you need. Because of limited resources, your local health or social services department may say they can only help people with the most serious needs. Or you may be promised help that fails to arrive.

If, for whatever reason, you cannot get the help you need, ask the person you are dealing with for an explanation. If you are not satisfied with what they say, or if you believe you have been treated unfairly, ask to speak to the manager. Explain what has happened and why you find it unacceptable. You could consider making a formal complaint.

Council (local authority) services

If you are unhappy about a service run by a council department, find out about the complaints procedure. Social services, for example, have a duty to deal properly and swiftly with complaints, and to explain the procedure to you. Contact your social services office and ask how the procedure works.

The first stage will be for you to complain informally. If you are not satisfied with the result, you may decide to make a formal complaint – this must be in writing.

If you have a complaint about any council service, you can also speak to your local councillor or to the councillor who is chairperson of the committee that runs the service. Your council's information service can tell you how to contact them.

Note Since March 1997, local authorities can take their own resources into account when deciding whether someone has a need for a service under the Chronically Sick and Disabled Persons Act 1970, and which services they will then arrange or provide. Services cannot be withdrawn or reduced until the person's care needs have been assessed (or reassessed) against revised eligibility criteria. Any reduction in, withdrawal of, or refusal to provide services must not leave individuals at severe physical risk.

Health services

If you are not happy with services provided by the NHS, contact your Community Health Council or Health Council in Scotland (in the phone book). This is an independent watchdog organisation which can give advice about any aspect of getting NHS services.

Respite care

Carers need a break from caring to reduce stress, stay healthy and keep going. You need to arrange some sort of break at least one day a week, if you can. See Chapter 6 (p 60) for more information.

Aids, appliances and adaptations

If your relative is disabled, an occupational therapist should assess his needs and make recommendations about adaptations to the home and about aids and appliances that could help increase independence. Ask the GP or social services if an occupational therapist's assessment isn't arranged.

People on low income can get help with the cost of adaptations. Contact social services or the local authority housing/environmental health department for information. The housing/environmental health department is responsible for the Home Repair Assistance Grant (not available in Scotland) and the Disabled Facilities Grant, and for adapting council housing. Charities are another possible source of help. Age Concern England has Factsheets dealing with repairs to the home.

Aids and appliances are generally supplied free or for a small fee by social services or the hospital. The Red Cross also lends or hires equipment such as wheelchairs, commodes and air-rings. You can buy aids and equipment, but this is expensive. Hire or borrow first, if you can, as people often abandon gadgets after using them only a few times. Get advice on aids and appliances from your local Disabled Living Centre or from the Disabled Living Foundation.

Changing needs

Both your needs and your relative's are likely to change over time. Your relative may become ill or need more care, or you may realise that something was overlooked in the original assessment. Your own health may get worse, and caring for someone for a long time is very wearing. If you need more help or support, you are entitled to ask social services for a reassessment of needs. Remember to give as much information as possible about what has changed, and what would help.

Benefits

Benefits your relative might be entitled to

Sick and disabled people and their carers are entitled to a range of social security benefits. A stroke can mean that family finances are turned upside down. If your relative has to give up work, or you have to give up work to care for him, there may be much less money coming into the household than before. It is worth making sure that you and your relative are getting all the welfare benefits that you are entitled to.

Some people feel reluctant to ask for financial help, but this is exactly what benefits are for: to protect people who, through no fault of their own, are unable to support themselves. If you are not sure whether your relative might be entitled to a benefit, you have nothing to lose by claiming – if you delay, you may lose out because a successful claim cannot be backdated.

The government office that deals with Social Security benefits is now called the Benefits Agency. The regulations about what you can get are complex, so it is well worth getting advice. Benefits Agency free helplines give confidential advice:

■ Benefit Enquiry Line Tel: 0800 88 22 00 – advice about benefits for people with disabilities and their carers.

Staff can help you work out which benefits you are entitled to, send out information and claim forms, and help you fill in a claim form over the phone. You can also get independent advice and help with completing claim forms from the Citizens Advice Bureau, your council's welfare rights/benefits advice service, or your local centre for the unemployed.

For more *i*nformation

❶ Leaflet FB2 *Which benefit?* – a guide to Social Security and NHS benefits.

❶ Leaflet FB31 *Caring for someone* – advice on benefits and other kinds of help available to carers.

101

- *ℹ* Leaflet API *A helping hand* – explains how to help someone with a disability to claim the benefits due to them.

- *ℹ* Leaflet FB28 *Sick or disabled?* – a guide to benefits if you're sick or disabled for a few days or more.

- *ℹ* Leaflet IB201 *Incapacity Benefit* – a guide to the new benefit that has replaced Sickness Benefit and Invalidity Benefit.

- *ℹ* Leaflet DS702 *Attendance allowance* – explains the benefit available to people over 65 who need help with personal care because of illness or disability.

- *ℹ* Leaflet DS704 *Disability Living Allowance* – information on the benefit available to people under 66 who need help with personal care or with getting around.

- *ℹ* Leaflet DS703 *Disability Working Allowance* – explains the benefit for disabled people in work.

- *ℹ* Leaflet IS50 *Income Support. Help if you live in a residential care home or nursing home* – information on benefits for people living in private sector homes.

You can get leaflets by phoning the helplines, or from the post office or Benefits Agency/Social Security office, or by post from BA Distribution and Storage Centre, Manchester Road, Heywood, Lancashire OL10 2PZ.

Independent Living Fund

The Independent Living Fund (ILF) is not strictly speaking a welfare benefit – it is a charitable fund set up by the Government for people who are so severely disabled that they would otherwise have to go into a residential home, but who would prefer to live in a place of their own with support. The ILF covers the cost of care for the person to live at home, up to a total of £500 per week, but the social services department must provide at least the first £200 per week of care services.

People cannot usually apply to the ILF themselves. The social services department has to apply on their behalf, and has to show that they are providing £200 worth of services.

To get help from the ILF someone must:

■ be aged 16–65;
■ be so severely disabled that they qualify for the highest level of the care component of the Disability Living Allowance;
■ be living alone or with someone who is not able to look after them;
■ be on Income Support, or have an income so low that it does not cover the cost of their care;
■ have savings of less than £8,000.

Money from the ILF does not affect any other benefits in any way. It is classed as a gift from a charitable trust, and it is not counted as income when Income Support is assessed.

Direct payments

Since April 1997 it has been possible for local authorities to give people money instead of (or as well as) services. These are known as direct payments. Individuals may use this money to organise and buy the care they have been assessed as needing by the local authority. Some services are excluded from direct payments – in particular, those services provided by a close relative living in the same household or elsewhere (except in exceptional circumstances). At present older people who are over 65 cannot receive direct payments. If you are the carer of an older person who has been assessed by the local authority as needing care services in their own home, and would prefer to organise and buy it themselves, contact Age Concern England.

For more *i*nformation

ℹ *Living with Stroke* by Paul King, published by Manchester University Press, 1990. This book has very helpful chapters on the emotional and psychological aspects of stroke. (Out of print, but may be available from a library.)

ⓘ *Directory for Disabled People* by Ann Darnborough and Derek Kinrade, published by Woodhead-Faulkner, 1995. Detailed information on rights, benefits, employment, sport, holidays etc.

ⓘ From the Stroke Association:

Booklet S5 *Understanding stroke illness*

Booklet S7 Stroke – *A handbook for the patient's family*

Booklet S9 *Psychological effects of stroke – A guide for the carer*

Leaflet S10 *On leaving hospital after a stroke*

Booklet S13 *Stroke and incontinence*

Leaflet S14 *How occupational therapy helps stroke patients*

Leaflet S16 *Sex after stroke illness*

Leaflet S18 *Swallowing difficulties after stroke*

Booklet S19 *Stroke and wheelchairs*

Booklet S20 *Stroke in young adults*

Leaflet S21 *Physiotherapy and strokes*

ⓘ From Age Concern England:

Factsheet 6 *Finding help at home*

Factsheet 10 *Local authority charging procedures for residential and nursing home care*

Factsheet 13 *Older home owners: financial help with repairs and adaptations*

Factsheet 29 *Finding residential and nursing home accommodation*

Factsheet 41 *Local authority assessments for community care services*

8 Rehabilitation

Rehabilitation builds on our natural attempts to overcome our disabilities. Its purpose is to help a disabled person regain as much ability and independence as possible. Its success depends on the extent of the stroke, the quality of the professional help and the motivation of the person involved. Carers have a crucial role in underpinning this motivation: their support can do much to help the success of the therapy.

Rehabilitation is a key stage in the recovery from stroke. If successful, it can enable the individual to achieve a more fulfilling and independent future than would otherwise be possible. It is well worth finding out as much as possible about how rehabilitation can help your relative. This chapter guides you through the problems and opportunities it may present.

Graham

'It takes time but I'm always moving forward, building on what I've done before.'

'The most important thing is to stop looking back at the past through rose-tinted spectacles and to learn to look forward to the future.

'I looked at my recovery as a ten-year project; I'm five years down the road now and I'm still improving. My aim is to remove the last tell-tale signs – the stroke walk and the stiffness in my hand. I set myself targets along the way and then I feel like I am achieving something. It takes time but I'm always moving forward, building on what I've done before.

'It's easy to get downhearted. It's sometimes hard to take the unthinking comments of others. I get angry, I can't cope with criticism, especially from someone who couldn't lace my boots before. But you have to get over it – I think to myself it shows their incompetence not mine. And there is so much to hope for, there is so much happening in the treatment of stroke now. New therapies come along all the time, offering new hope. We've got a file on new developments at the stroke club and we get doctors and therapists to come and talk to us regularly. We keep ourselves well informed.'

What you can do to help your relative's rehabilitation

How much someone is affected by a stroke depends on the severity of the stroke and the determination to overcome it. As with all diseases, the will to get better is important in determining the final outcome. There are many examples of people with massive strokes making remarkable recoveries and of people with relatively minor strokes giving up and turning their faces to the wall. With stroke, positive thought is essential: one of the most helpful things you can do as a carer is to nurture positive thinking in your relative. Your attitude to the illness and the expectations of recovery can make a real difference.

Before you can get your relative to think positively, you need to have a positive frame of mind yourself. A powerful way of motivating yourself is to recognise the difference that you can make to your relative's recovery. The professional help of therapists and doctors in rehabilitating your relative is, of course, essential but their resources are limited. Much of the practical work of rehabilitation has to be carried out at home. By creating an atmosphere that encourages striving and independence, and by ensuring that your relative does her exercises regularly, you will create the conditions for the best possible recovery.

Anyone who is disabled learns new ways to walk or talk. The aim of rehabilitation is to help this process, enabling people to be as independent as possible. You can help your relative do this by:

- motivating her;
- arranging a professional diagnosis and programme of treatment for her problems;
- setting up a daily routine that promotes rehabilitation;
- encouraging her to be active.

Motivating your relative

Overcoming the disabilities caused by stroke is one of the most difficult things anyone can do. As with any difficulty, success in overcoming it depends on motivation. With stroke the ability to motivate ourselves is often undermined. Our sense of self is damaged, our role in the family and society is often taken away, our body no longer does what we want it to and our mental faculties are disrupted; depression and anxiety are common states of mind. Carers can help to restore motivation. During the early stages of recovery the rapid progress often supplies its own motivation but when this starts to slow down, real help is needed to continue improving.

Motivating your relative requires understanding of the task she faces. The better you understand the damage caused to her physical and mental abilities, the more insight you will have into her difficulties. This will also help you to maintain your own morale as you will be able to appreciate the effort that your relative puts into apparently simple tasks. You can find out about your relative's stroke by talking to the doctors and therapists, by reading books, leaflets and other publications, by talking to the members of other families who have experience of stroke and by using the information and advisory services of organisations such as the Stroke Association.

It is important to show your relative that she still matters to you and is a valued member of your family. Try to include her in the daily family routine, give her real responsibilities that she can handle. Involve her in all the family activities so that she feels she is contributing to the life of the family. Never talk about her as though she weren't there, and don't let other people do it either. If she has difficulty talking, explain to other people exactly what communication difficulties she has, and remind them not to shout at her as though she were deaf. Explain that just because people can't talk it doesn't mean they can't understand.

Encouraging your relative

Supporting your relative is a matter of fine judgement. On the one hand she needs to feel that you are caring and compassionate, on the other it is important not to cosset her into inactivity. For her own sake she must be encouraged to do as much as she possibly can. Remember: when you do something for your relative you are denying her the opportunity of learning to do it for herself. It may be quicker, but in the long term it is disabling.

Your relative may resent you always asking her to go that little bit further and will tell you so. Listen to her reasons and explore her anxieties; remember that especially in the early days she will tire quickly. If her objections are sound, work out a way of accommodating them. If they are not, you need to be firm and gently insistent that she carries on developing her abilities. You should expect to face resistance and resentment from your relative; your job is to overcome these and to replace them with motivation and co-operation.

You can help your relative and at the same time boost her confidence by breaking down big tasks into smaller ones that are achievable. For example, she won't feel able to go to the shops on her own before she can walk to the garden gate. By breaking tasks into small achievable targets you can make each practice session rewarding in itself. You also avoid the frustration and despair caused by asking your relative to do something she just can't do.

Maintain your relative's pride in her appearance

You can show your relative that you value her by helping her maintain her appearance. Make sure that her personal hygiene is kept up to the old standards, that she is well groomed, that she has her normal make-up, that her clothes are clean and neat. Make sure she has any aids such as hearing aids or glasses that she would have used before the stroke, and that if she uses dentures they still fit. Check that she is able to clean her teeth properly; if her face has been affected, check that food does not get lodged in the paralysed side. Make sure that her clothing is appropriate and will help her maintain modesty; trousers, for example, may be better than skirts for some exercises. Encourage her not to become overweight or, if she is overweight, to lose weight because excess weight discourages activity and makes it more difficult to regain movement.

Professional diagnosis and treatment

If your relative has communication difficulties or paralysis she will need to see an appropriate therapist. It is important for you, as her main carer, to accompany her to these meetings. This is because the therapist will explain to both of you the causes of your relative's problems and will show you how to help her to do the necessary exercises.

Speech and language problems

For difficulties with speech, understanding, reading or writing your relative needs to see a speech and language therapist. The therapist will diagnose your relative's problems by carrying out a series of tests; from these he or she will be able to explain what you and your relative can do to help her communicate more effectively. The therapist will also recommend exercises that could help. (Speech problems are discussed in Chapter 3.) Try to get as clear a picture as you can of what your relative's problems are. If the therapist uses unfamiliar words, ask for an explanation. You may also find an explanation in the Glossary in this book. Write down the speech therapist's explanation so you can refer to it in the future.

Speech therapy relies heavily on frequent short exercise sessions but also on reinforcing the skills throughout the day. Detailed advice on how to help your relative should be taken from the therapist, but common ground rules are:

■ Never assume that someone who has had a stroke can't understand.

■ Make sure that any hearing aids are used and are working.

■ Don't shout.

■ Speak slowly, in short sentences.

■ Allow your relative time to express herself.

■ Limit correction to set 'training' sessions; at other times pick up the misused word and say it back properly in a new sentence.

■ Similarly, if your relative uses single words, pick them up and put them in an appropriate sentence.

■ When your relative gets something right, tell her and give her praise.

■ Use gesture and mime to reinforce the meaning of your words.

■ Encourage her all the time.

■ If you don't understand, don't pretend that you do.

■ Remember that your relative may tire quickly.

The Stroke Association runs Dysphasic Support groups throughout England and Wales. These provide help in the home with speech and associated problems; they also run group sessions which help people rebuild confidence in their language skills. The Stroke Association publishes a leaflet, S2 *Learning to speak again*, which contains hints on helping someone who has communication difficulties. It also publishes a Word and Picture Chart which can be used to point at when someone can't speak. Action for Dysphasic Adults (ADA) also provides advice and support for dysphasic people and their families. Information can be obtained from Chest, Heart and Stroke, Scotland, and from Northern Ireland Chest, Heart and Stroke Association, who also run local support groups.

Paralysis problems

The physiotherapist and occupational therapist (OT) help people who have problems with paralysis. The exact demarcation between the two sets of therapists varies according to the hospital and health authority. Generally the physiotherapist deals with problems with movement – walking and use of the arm and hand – and the OT deals with problems in carrying out particular activities such as eating, grooming, cooking, using a keyboard and so on.

If your relative has communication or memory problems, mention them to the physiotherapist and OT. Otherwise the therapists may think your relative is being uncooperative when in fact she either doesn't understand or has forgotten what she has been asked to do.

These therapists will diagnose your relative's problems and devise a course of treatment. They will also assess what aids and equipment your relative needs and whether adaptations should be made to her home. The physiotherapist will explain to carers how to move their relative, how to minimise the effects of spasticity and what exercises can be done to improve her use of her limbs.

When doing exercises at home make sure that there are no mats or furniture to trip over, that the floors aren't slippery and that your relative is wearing appropriate clothing and footwear. Exercises should be short and frequent, and encouragement constant; criticism has no place.

General advice on how to help your relative regain mobility is contained in the books and leaflets listed at the end of the chapter, but for detailed advice you should consult her therapists. They will prescribe a programme of rehabilitation that is tailored to your relative's needs.

Arrange a daily routine

During rehabilitation your relative's 'job' is to recover her independence, so as far as possible construct the day around it. Plan the day around the exercise sessions, trips for therapy and trips to support groups. Exercise sessions work best if they are frequent and short, so ask the therapists for advice on how often to do them each day. Setting up a routine helps to ensure that exercises are done regularly; if you only do them when you feel like it they will often get missed.

The whole point of the therapy and exercises is to re-equip your relative for dealing with life. Set up a daily routine which makes use of the skills that your relative is learning in therapy. That way life and therapy reinforce each other. Encourage her throughout the day to communicate, move and manipulate things. As her skills and confidence develop, give her more and more household responsibilities. Remember that it is important for both of you to have social contact, so build in time during your week to have guests or to go visiting. Equally, it is important to enjoy your lives, so build in leisure activities and breaks for yourself.

Keep your relative active

Always try to encourage your relative to be active: the less active she is, the less active she will want to be. Also, the less active she is, the more likely she is to put on weight. Apart from certain heart conditions, rest has no particular role in the recovery from stroke. Encourage your relative to be active from the beginning. The more she gets out of shape, the harder she will have to work to get it back again. Make use of the sports facilities available to the disabled; find out what there is locally by contacting social services or the voluntary organisations for the disabled listed in Useful Addresses. The Chartered Society of Physiotherapy publishes leaflets on safe exercises for older people.

When rehabilitation ends

'At the stroke club, Diane told me how they stopped Harold's speech therapy dead without warning. I was shocked but when it happened to me a fortnight later, I was so glad I had been warned about it by Diane. I don't know how I would have coped if I hadn't had that conversation.'

When therapy ends is often a time of stress for the person who has had the stroke and for the carer. People often feel that they have been abandoned by the health service and think that the end of therapy sessions implies that the health professionals believe there is no further chance for recovery. The fact is that the time comes when the emphasis on improving recovery switches to adapting to the residual disability.

Therapy departments set themselves practical objectives with each patient because they have limited resources. Ending the treatment does not mean that your relative will not continue to improve. Neither is it the end of rehabilitation because, as we have seen, much rehabilitation takes place at home anyway. Also, you can continue to get support from voluntary organisations.

To reduce the stress of the end of therapy, talk about it to the therapists right from the start. Ask them what they hope to achieve and how long they think treatment will take. Then make arrangements to get support from voluntary organisations. Ask the therapists or your doctor about any local support groups, contact the Stroke Association to see if there is a Dysphasic Support scheme in your area and contact RADAR (Royal Association for Disability and Rehabilitation) or one of the other disability aid organisations listed in the Useful Addresses section for information and advice.

If you or your relative feel depression or despair at the end of therapy, talk to someone about it – your family, friends, stroke group, local support groups or GP. Try to regard the end of therapy as a milestone on the road to recovery. Re-read the advice in Chapter 7 on dealing with depression and anxiety. If you feel that your relative really needs to continue with therapy and that she is not receiving the treatment she is entitled to, contact your Community Health Council and ask them to do something about it.

For more *i*nformation

ℹ *Living with Stroke* by Paul King, published by Manchester University Press. (Out of print, but may be available in libraries.)

ⓘ *Stroke* by Dr RM Young – especially the two chapters 'Learning to walk again' and 'Problems of communication'; published by David and Charles.

ⓘ Stroke Association publications:

Leaflet S2 *Learning to speak again*

Booklet S5 *Understanding stroke illness*

Booklet S7 *Stroke – a handbook for the patient's family*

Leaflet S14 *How occupational therapy helps stroke patients*

Leaflet S21 *Physiotherapy and strokes*

Booklet S25 *Cognitive problems following stroke, including a glossary of terms*

9 Keeping healthy: life after stroke

Most of this book has been about overcoming past illness and coming to terms with the present. This chapter is about looking forward to the future. It's about keeping healthy and positive living.

Luke

'I've just done a plan of the garden and its colours at different seasons.'

'Recovering from stroke I developed parts of my character that I had neglected before.

'I'd always promised myself that I would get to grips with computers, and in fact I had bought one before my stroke but never had the time to really use it. Then I had my stroke. I couldn't use my right hand, my speech came out like a drunken voice simulator and I used to cry with frustration at not being able to communicate with people. And so I switched on my computer, I keyed in everything with my left hand, corrected it, spell-checked it and finally printed a perfect page. That page was a triumph, and from that I went on to write about everything. I wrote about my experience of stroke, I wrote for my church magazine and I do the newsletter for the stroke group. I also keep a diary every day on it. I still use mainly my left hand, although I can use my right for simple things like the space bar and the return key.

'The other thing I did was get a graphics package – not an expensive one – and now I spend a lot of time doing cartoons and illustrations, or just playing around on it. I've just done a plan of the garden and its colours at different seasons. I think it's the artistic side of my brain taking over now my analytical side isn't so dominant. I listen to a lot more music too.'

Keeping healthy

After a stroke many people worry about having another. If your relative worries about this, point out that the overwhelming majority (nine out of ten) of people who have had a stroke will not have another one in the next year. Your relative does have a slightly increased risk of stroke but has a much greater risk of death from arterial and heart disease. Healthy living after stroke depends on following general advice on exercise, weight and what we eat, and taking care of our heart and arteries.

Have regular health check-ups

Arrange for your relative to see his GP on a regular basis after his stroke, say once a year. Discuss how often with his GP, who may want to see him sooner if he is on medication. Most people who have a stroke are over 65 and half are over 75. If your relative is elderly, it makes sense to have a regular check-up anyway. If your relative is disabled, some of his problems may get worse as he gets older, and these too need reassessing on a regular basis.

Keeping in good health

There are a few aspects of health that need special attention after stroke:

Constipation Some people suffer from constipation after stroke. This is often the result of inactivity and insufficient fibre in the diet. So encourage your relative to be more active and encourage him to eat a healthier diet that contains more fibre. Also make sure he drinks enough water. If the problem persists, he should see his GP.

Anxiety and depression are common after a stroke. If your relative gets locked into either of these mental states, get help (see p 80).

Central post-stroke pain is a burning, shooting and throbbing pain that develops some time after the stroke and is not eased by painkillers. It occurs in about 2 per cent of people who have had a stroke, usually in those under 60. Many GPs are not aware of the condition, which can be treated. A free leaflet, S23 *Central post-stroke pain*, is available from the Stroke Association. They also publish another leaflet on this specifically for GPs.

Epilepsy Sometimes people develop epilepsy after stroke, due to the scarring of brain tissue. This can be treated by drugs. If your relative develops fits, make sure he sees his GP. The Stroke Association publishes a leaflet on epilepsy: S15 *Epilepsy after stroke*.

High blood pressure (hypertension) is one of the contributory causes of stroke. It is important that it be reduced because the closer blood pressure is to normal the less the risk of stroke. If your relative has high blood pressure, it is important that he takes medication for it and that he has it checked on a regular basis.

Heart disease As we have seen, people who have had a stroke are more likely to die from heart disease than from another stroke. After the stroke your relative should have had a thorough examination of his heart and arteries. The doctor may have prescribed medication and will have given advice on diet and exercise. It is important for your relative's health that he follows these recommendations.

Preventative medication Your relative may have been prescribed medicines after his stroke to reduce the risk of clots forming. Aspirin and warfarin are common examples. Make sure your relative takes his doses regularly.

Smoking The simple advice is: don't – it will kill you. It damages the heart, arteries and lungs, reduces the ability of the blood to carry oxygen, causes cancer and is addictive. The organisation Quit will give advice on stopping smoking.

117

Alcohol There is no reason to stop drinking alcohol so long as it is drunk in moderation. Excessive drinking can increase blood pressure. Men should not drink more than three units of alcohol a day, or women two units. A unit is the amount of alcohol in half a pint of beer or a glass of wine.

Looking to the future: healthy, positive living

You can encourage your relative to take an optimistic attitude to the future by persuading him that his actions affect his future health. By taking steps to improve his future health he will increase his sense of control over his own life, and this in itself will improve his outlook and his sense of well-being. There is no magic formula in this: most of us already know what we ought to be doing, it's just a question of doing it. There is one advantage that someone getting over a stroke generally has and that is time. Time to eat well, keep fit and develop a social life. Below are some suggestions for a healthy life-style.

Food

Your relative needs a well balanced diet that will keep him at the right weight for his height and body type. Among older people, problems arise from both over-eating and under-eating, so look out for both possibilities.

Avoid excess sugar and fats (see 'Eating too much fat' in Chapter 1), eat plenty of fibre (vegetables, fresh fruit and whole grain cereals) and avoid excess salt. Avoid highly processed foods – they are usually high in fat and sugar or salt, and low in fibre. Encourage your relative to experiment with different foods. If he can, get him involved in the preparation and cooking.

For free advice on healthy eating, phone the Health Information Service on freephone 0800 66 55 44.

Exercise

Keeping fit is essential for good health. It will help to keep your relative's weight down and help him to keep active. Not only will exercise improve his muscles, heart and lungs – it will also put him in a better frame of mind. The exercise does not have to be especially vigorous to be beneficial, a regular walk each day is often enough. Many disabled people find swimming particularly enjoyable because the buoyancy gives them a sense of freedom. If your relative has high blood pressure, he should talk to his GP before starting vigorous exercise.

For free advice on keeping fit, phone the Health Information Service on freephone 0800 66 55 44.

Weight control

Excess weight makes it difficult to keep active, and can cause heart and other health problems. If your relative is overweight, he should reduce his calorie intake and increase his activity. Diets that reduce weight suddenly do not work in the long run and can be harmful to health. Your GP will advise you how to reduce weight safely. Alternatively, the practice nurse or a dietician can help.

Free advice on weight reduction is given by the Health Information Service on freephone 0800 66 55 44.

Sex

Sex is important in many relationships as a way of demonstrating love and drawing the partners closer together. For the person who has had a stroke it can be a powerful demonstration that his partner still loves him. Generally there is no medical reason for giving up sex after stroke but there may be physical or psychological problems that make sex difficult. Usually these difficulties can be overcome, given good advice and the willingness of both partners. See the section on sex in Chapter 7.

Leisure

Leisure activities are essential for a fulfilling life. They bring us into contact with other people, and give us something to look forward to and to talk about afterwards. If disabilities restrict some opportunities, support groups, voluntary organisations and local authorities open up others. Holiday guides for disabled people and their carers are available from Holiday Care Service. RADAR provides information about holidays and other leisure activities, and the Stroke Association quarterly magazine *Stroke News* has listings of leisure activities.

Driving

The return to driving is an important psychological step for many people who have had a stroke. Driving in our society is associated with independence and adulthood. The law requires that anyone who has had a stroke or a TIA must inform the Driver and Vehicle Licensing Agency (DVLA). The DVLA will make medical enquiries and after a month will write to you saying whether you may resume driving or not. If after a month you have not heard from DVLA, you must see your own doctor; if he or she agrees, you can return to driving. You must also inform your insurance company that you have had a stroke.

The Stroke Association publishes an excellent booklet on returning to driving: S22 *Driving after stroke*.

Employment

Employment is important for financial reasons, and for the sense of identity, self-worth and social contact it gives. Most people who have a stroke are past retiring age, but, for those who can, returning to work gives a boost to their self-confidence and optimism about the future.

The return to work, even if for only a few days a week, marks a major stage in the process of recovery. It may involve a period of retraining and may place an emotional and physical strain on your relative. Encourage him in his efforts to return to work, and when he is disheartened remind him of the progress he has already made. The effort is well worth it both for your relative and for yourself: it will encourage you both to start looking to the future rather than the past.

If your relative wishes to return to work and his doctor agrees, his first course of action should be to contact his former employer to discuss the possibilities of returning to his former job. If there are specific problems, an occupational therapist may be able to suggest ways of reorganising the task or the use of specialised aids that will overcome the difficulties.

The next person to contact is the Disablement Employment Advisor (DEA) at your relative's local Employment Service Jobcentre. The DEA will help him decide a course of action, which may be through further assessment by a Placement, Assessment and Counselling Team (PACT) or through suitable employment or training. PACTs are based locally and they advise and counsel on returning to work. They will draw up an action plan with your relative for his return to work.

The DEA can also advise your relative on the Employment Service Special Schemes. These are a range of schemes that can provide special aids, travel to work grants and adaptations to premises and equipment to enable disabled people to return to work. To qualify for one of these special schemes your relative may need to be registered under the Disabled Persons (Employment) Act 1944. This Act requires all employers of more than 20 people to have a minimum 3 per cent quota of its workforce registered disabled people.

Further advice on return to work can be obtained from the Stroke Association or Opportunities for Jobs. The Stroke Association booklet S20 *Stroke in younger adults* also provides excellent advice.

Life after stroke for the carer

It is equally important for you, the carer, to look after your own health and to be positive about the future. We saw in Chapter 6 that it is important for carers to have breaks from caring and to maintain interests of their own. Caring imposes its own strains on your health, so it is important that you pay attention to your own needs and, if you have problems, to seek help early.

As you build up your support networks and your life starts to assume a more orderly routine, it is important to look to the future. It may be possible to resume employment if you've not already retired or, if you have, to pick up activities that you were involved in before your relative's stroke. Develop new interests and new friendships. You may enjoy holidays with your relative but also consider going away without him. Get other family members or friends to provide the care while you are away, or make use of the respite services mentioned in Chapter 6. You may feel guilty about doing this but don't. The happier you are the happier you will be able to make your relative.

For more *i*nformation

i Stroke Association publications:

Leaflet S15 *Epilepsy after stroke*

Booklet S22 *Driving after stroke*

Leaflet S23 *Central post-stroke pain*

Useful addresses

Action for Dysphasic Adults (ADA)
Information, support and advice
for dysphasic adults and their
families. Local branches run
support and social groups.

1 Royal Street
London SE1 7LL
Tel: 0171-261 9572

**Action on Smoking and Health
(ASH)**
Medical charity that campaigns
to alert the public to the dangers
of smoking Publishes a range of
ASH Factsheets. Has local groups
throughout England.

16 Fitzhardinge Street
London W1H 9PL
Tel: 0171-224 0743

**Alzheimer Scotland – Action on
Dementia**
Information, support and advice
about dementia for people in
Scotland.

22 Drumsheugh Gardens
Edinburgh EH3 7RN
Office: 0131-243 1453
24-hour helpline:
0800 317 817

Alzheimer's Disease Society
Information, support and advice
about caring for someone with
Alzheimer's disease.

Gordon House
10 Greencoat Place
London SW1P 1PH
Tel: 0171-306 0606
Fax: 0171-306 0808

WALES
**Heol Don Resource Centre for
the Elderly**

Heol Don
Whitchurch
Cardiff CF4 2XG
Tel: 01222 521872

Association of Charity Officers
Advice on how to find out about charities that could help you.

Beechwood House
Wyllyotts Close
Potters Bar
Herts EN6 2HN
Tel: 01707 651777

Association of Crossroads Care Attendant Schemes
See Crossroads Care

Benefits Agency
Advice about state benefits for people with disabilities and their carers.

Benefit Enquiry Line:
0800 88 22 00

BA Distribution and Storage Centre
For information leaflets about the various state benefits.

Manchester Road
Heywood
Lancashire OL10 2PZ

British Association for Counselling
To find out about counselling services in your area.

1 Regent Place
Rugby
Warwickshire CV21 2PJ
Tel: 01788 578328/9

British Heart Foundation
Information about all aspects of heart disease.

14 Fitzhardinge Street
London W1H 4DH
Tel: 0171-935 0185

British Lung Foundation
Information about all aspects of lung disease.

78 Hatton Garden
London EC1N 8JR
Tel: 0171-831 5831

British Red Cross
Can lend or hire home aids for disabled people. Local branches in many cities.

9 Grosvenor Crescent
London SW1X 7EJ
Tel: 0171-235 5454

Calibre
Free audio cassette library for blind people.

Aylesbury
Buckingham HP22 5XQ
Tel: 01296 432339/81211

Care Alternatives – Care for the Elderly
A private agency that provides care for elderly people in their own homes. Mainly London area but can arrange live-in care nationwide.

206 Worple Road
London SW20 8PW
Tel: 0181-946 8202

Care and Repair Ltd
Advice about home repairs and improvements.

Castle House
Kirtley Drive
Nottingham NG7 1LD
Tel: 0115 979 9091

Carematch
Computerised information about residential care for people with physical disabilities.

286 Camden Road
London N7 OBJ
Tel: 0171-609 9966

Carers National Association
Information and advice if you are caring for someone. Can put you in touch with other carers and carers' groups in your area.

20–25 Glasshouse Yard
London EC1A 4JS
Tel: 0171-490 8818
(Adviceline:
0171-490 8898
1–4pm weekdays)

LONDON REGION

5 Chalton Street
London NW1 1JD
Tel: 0171-383 3460

SCOTLAND

3rd Floor
162 Buchanan Street
Glasgow G1 2LL
Tel: 0141-333 9495

NORTH OF ENGLAND

Humphrey Booth Institute
Ladywell Hospital
Eccles New Road
Salford M5 2AA
Tel: 0161-707 8600

CARERS NATIONAL ASSOCIATION IN WALES

Pant Glas Industrial Estate
Bedwas
Newport
Gwent NP1 8DR
Tel: 01222 880176

125

3rd Floor
113 University Street
Belfast BT7 1HP
Tel: 01232 439843

Chest, Heart and Stroke Association
See Stroke Association, British Heart Foundation *and* British Lung Foundation

Chest, Heart and Stroke Scotland

65 North Castle Street
Edinburgh EH2 3LT
Tel: 0131-225 6963

Northern Ireland Chest, Heart and Stroke Association

21 Dublin Road
Belfast BT2 7FJ
Tel: 01232 320184

Citizens Advice Bureau
For advice on legal, financial and consumer matters. A good place to turn to if you don't know where to go for help or advice on any subject.

Listed in local telephone directories or in *Yellow Pages* under social service and welfare organisations. Other local advice centres may also be listed.

Community Health Council (Health Council in Scotland)
For enquiries or complaints about any aspect of the NHS in your area.

See the local telephone directory for your area (sometimes listed under Health Authority).

Continence Foundation
Advice and information about whom to contact with incontinence problems.

The Basement
2 Doughty Street
London WC1N 2PH
Tel: 0171-404 6875

Counsel and Care
Advice for elderly people and their families; can sometimes give grants to help people remain at home or to return to their home.

Lower Ground Floor
Twyman House
16 Bonny Street
London NW1 9PG
Tel: 0171-485 1566

Court of Protection
*If you need Power of Attorney to
take over the affairs of someone
who is mentally incapable.*

Public Trust Office
Protection Division
Stewart House
24 Kingsway
London WC2B 6JX
Tel: 0171-664 7300

Crossroads Care
*For a care attendant to come
into your home and look after
your relative.*

10 Regent Place
Rugby
Warwickshire CV21 2PN
Tel: 01788 573653

CRUSE – Bereavement Care
*Comfort in bereavement. Can
put you in touch with people in
your area.*

126 Sheen Road
Richmond
Surrey TW9 1UR
Tel: 0181-940 4818/9047

**Department of Social Security
(DSS)**
*Formerly DHSS. Welfare rights
and benefits section is called the
Benefits Agency.*

See your local telephone
directory.

**DIAL UK (Disablement
Information and Advice Lines)**
*Information and advice for people
with disabilities. Can put you in
touch with local contacts.*

Park Lodge
St Catherine's Hospital
Tickhill Road
Balby
Doncaster DN4 8QN
Tel: 01302 310123

**Disability Alliance Education
and Research Association**
*Campaigning for a better deal
for people with disabilities;
information about welfare benefits.*

1st Floor East
Universal House
88–94 Wentworth Street
London E1 7SA
Tel: 0171-247 8776
Welfare rights enquiries:
0171-247 8763

Disability Law Service
*Free legal advice for disabled
people and their families.*

2nd Floor
49–51 Bedford Row
London WC1R 4LR
Tel: 0171-831 8031/7740

Disabled Drivers' Association
*Information and advice for
disabled drivers.*

National HQ
Ashwellthorpe Hall
Norwich
Norfolk NR16 lEX
Tel: 01508 489 449

Disabled Drivers' Motor Club
*Information and advice about
mobility problems for disabled
people, whether they are drivers
or passengers.*

Cottingham Way
Thrapston
Northants NN14 4PL
Tel: 01832 734724

Disabled Living Centres Council
*Can tell you where your nearest
Disabled Living Centre is, where
you can see and try out aids
and equipment.*

286 Camden Road
London N7 OBJ
Tel: 0171-700 1707

Disabled Living Foundation
*Information about aids to help
you cope with a disability.*

380–384 Harrow Road
London W9 2HU
Tel: 0171-289 6111

Disability Scotland
*National organisation for
information on all non-medical
aspects of disability.*

Princes House
5 Shandwick Place
Edinburgh EH2 4RG
Tel: 0131-229 8632
(voice and textphone)

Disability Wales
*National association of disability
groups working to promote the
rights, recognition and support
of all disabled people in Wales.*

Llys Ifor
Crescent Road
Caerphilly CF83 1XL
Tel: 01222 887325

Elderly Accommodation Council
*Computerised information about
all forms of accommodation for
older people, including nursing
homes and hospices, and advice
on top-up funding.*

46a Chiswick High Road
London W4 1SZ
Tel: 0181-995 8320/
742 1182

Forces Help Society
Now merged with SSAFA.

Greater London Association for Disabled People (GLAD)
Information for disabled people in the London area.

336 Brixton Road
London SW9 7AA
Tel: 0171-274 0107

Headway (National Head Injuries Association)
For people who are disabled physically or mentally as a result of a head injury, and their carers.

7 King Edward Court
King Edward Street
Nottingham NG1 lEW
Tel: 0115 912 1000

Health Information Service
Advice on healthy eating, keeping fit and weight reduction.

Tel: 0800 66 55 44

Help the Aged
Advice and information for older people and their families.

16–18 St James's Walk
London EC1R OBE
Tel: 0171–253 0253
Winter Warmth
Hotline/Seniorline:
0800 650 065

Holiday Care Service
Free information and advice about holidays for elderly or disabled people and their carers.

2nd Floor
Imperial Buildings
Victoria Road
Horley
Surrey RH6 7PZ
Tel: 01293 771500

Incontinence Information Helpline
Information and advice about managing incontinence, and how to contact your nearest continence adviser.

Tel: 0191-213 0050

Jewish Care
Social care, personal support, residential homes for Jewish people.

Stuart Young House
221 Golders Green Road
London NW11 9DQ
Tel: 0181-458 3282

John Grooms Association for Disabled People
Residential, respite and holiday accommodation.

50 Scrutton Street
London EC2A 4PH
Tel: 0171-452 2000

129

Leonard Cheshire Foundation
Residential homes and home care attendants for disabled people.

26–29 Maunsel Street
London SW1P 2QN
Tel: 0171-828 1822

London Accessible Transport Unit (LATU)
Advice about transport for disabled people in the London area.

Policy Unit
Civic Centre
Lampton Road
Hounslow TW3 4DN
Tel: 0181-814 2891

Marriage Counselling Scotland
Counselling and help with difficult relationships.

105 Hanover Street
Edinburgh EH2 1DJ
Tel: 0131-225 5006

Mobility Advice and Vehicle Information Service (MAVIS)
Advice for disabled car drivers.

O Wing
Macadam Avenue
Old Wokingham Road
Crowthorne
Berks RG45 6XD
Tel: 01344 661000

Motability
Cars and wheelchairs for disabled people.

Goodman House
Station Approach
Harlow
Essex CM20 2ET
Tel: 01279 635666

National Association of Bereavement Services
Information about bereavement and loss counselling services in your area.

20 Norton Folgate
London E1 6DB
Tel: 0171-247 1080
(24-hour answerphone)

National Association of Councils for Voluntary Service
Can tell you how to find your local CVS, which puts volunteers in touch with people needing help.

3rd Floor
Arundel Court
177 Arundel Street
Sheffield S1 2NU
Tel: 0114 278 6636

National Association of Funeral Directors
Offers code of conduct and a simple service for a basic funeral.

618 Warwick Road
Solihull B91 1AA
Tel: 0121-711 1343

National Council for Voluntary Organisations (NCVO)
Information about voluntary organisations in your locality that could be a source of help.

Regents Wharf
8 All Saints Street
London N1 9RL
Tel: 0171-713 6161

National Head Injuries Association
See Headway

Opportunities for Jobs
Advice about returning to work.

Tel: 0181-235 0500

ParentAbility
Provides a contact register, resource list, helpline and a link service to help professionals caring for parents with disabilities.

National Childbirth Trust
Alexander House
Oldham Terrace
London W3 6NH
Tel: 0181-992 8637

Pensions Advisory Service
For queries and problems to do with occupational pensions.

11 Belgrave Road
London SW1V 1RB
Tel: 0171-233 8080

Quit
National charity helping smokers to stop smoking. Provides public and workplace courses and gives help to health professionals, GPs and the media. Runs 'Quitline', which smokers can ring for advice, information packs and details of local support groups.

Victory House
170 Tottenham Court Road
London W1P OHA
Tel: 0171-487 3000

RADAR (Royal Association for Disability and Rehabilitation)
Information about aids and mobility, holidays, sport and leisure for disabled people.

Unit 12
City Forum
250 City Road
London EC1V 8AF
Tel: 0171-250 3222

Registered Nursing Homes Association
Information about registered nursing homes in your area.

Calthorpe House
Hagley Road
Edgbaston
Birmingham B16 8QY
Tel: 0121-454 2511

Relate (formerly National Marriage Guidance Council)
Counselling and help with difficult relationships; many local branches.

Herbert Gray College
Little Church Street
Rugby
Warwickshire CV21 3AP
Tel: 01788 573241/
560811

Relatives' Association
Support and advice for the relatives of people in a residential or nursing home or hospital long term.

5 Tavistock Place
London WC1H 9SS
Tel: 0171-916 6055/
0181-201 9153

Samaritans
Someone to talk to if you are in despair.

See your local telephone directory.

Scope (formerly Spastics Society)
Provides help, advice and practical resources to people with cerebral palsy, their parents and carers.

12 Park Crescent
London WIN 4EQ
Tel: 0171-636 5020

Scottish Association for Mental Health
Information about services in Scotland for people with mental health problems.

Cumbrae House
15 Carlton Court
Glasgow G5 9JP
Tel: 0141-568 7000

Scottish Council for Voluntary Organisations
For information about voluntary organisations and councils for voluntary service in Scotland.

18–19 Claremont Crescent
Edinburgh EH7 4QD
Tel: 0131-556 3882

Self-Help Team
Information about self-help groups.

20 Pelham Road
Nottingham NG5 1AP
Tel: 0115-969 1212

Shaftesbury Society
Sheltered housing for older people.

16 Kingston Road
London SW19 1JZ
Tel: 0181-239 5555

Soldiers, Sailors and Airmen Family Association (SSAFA)
Help for service or ex-service men and women and their families.

19 Queen Elizabeth Street
London SE1 2LP
Tel: 0171-403 8783/
962 9696

SPOD (Association to Aid the Sexual and Personal Relationships of People with a Disability)
Telephone counselling Monday and Wednesday 1.30–4.30pm, and Tuesday and Thursday 10.30am–1.30pm.

286 Camden Road
London N7 OBJ
Tel: 0171-607 8851

Standing Conference of Ethnic Minority Senior Citizens
Information, support and advice for older people from ethnic minorities, and their families.

5 Westminster Bridge Road
London SE1 7XW
Tel: 0171-928 0095

Stroke Association
Information and advice if you are caring for someone who has had a stroke. See also Chest, Heart and Stroke Scotland, Northern Ireland Chest, Heart and Stroke Association.

123–127 Whitecross Street
London EC1Y 8JJ
Tel: 0171-490 7999
(1–3.55pm)

Tripscope
Free information and advice about travel and transport for disabled and older people.

The Courtyard
Evelyn Road
London W4 5JL
Tel/Textphone:
0345 585641

United Kingdom Home Care Association
For information about organisations providing home care in your area.

42B Banstead Road
Carshalton
Surrey SM5 3NW
Tel: 0181-288 1551

Women's Royal Voluntary Service
Provide meals at home for ill and disabled people in some areas.

Milton Hill House
Milton Hill
Abingdon
Oxfordshire
Tel: 01235 442900

Glossary

Aneurysm localised ballooning of an artery

Aorta the main artery from the heart that supplies blood to the rest of the body

Aphasia the loss of the ability to use language properly (see p 36)

Apraxia the loss of the ability to initiate or sequence the series of muscle movements necessary to pronounce a word or perform a learnt action (see p 36)

Arteries tubes that carry the blood from the heart to the rest of the body. *See also* Veins

Arteriosclerosis hardening of the arteries. Happens chiefly in old age

Atheroma narrowing of the arteries by build-up of fat, cholesterol and other deposits

Atherosclerosis narrowing of the arteries by the laying down of fats, cholesterol and other substances, which reduces the flow of blood and promotes the formation of clots. It is a major cause of death through stroke and heart disease

Atrial fibrillation irregular heart rhythm

Capillaries small blood vessels

Carotid angiogram a test that reveals any blockages in the carotid arteries (see p 23)

Carotid arteries two arteries, one running up each side of the neck. Each artery splits into an internal carotid artery, which supplies blood to the brain, and an external carotid artery which supplies the outside of the head – the throat, face and scalp. Carotid comes from the Greek word meaning 'to stupefy', because the arteries are squeezed in strangling. *Atherosclerosis* of the internal carotid is a common cause of stroke

Cerebral of the brain, from the Latin *cerebrum* meaning the brain

Cerebral embolism a blood clot in the brain that has travelled there from somewhere else

Cerebral haemorrhage bleeding into the brain from a burst artery

Cerebral thrombosis blockage of an artery supplying the brain

Contractures deformities in the joints of paralysed limbs that prevent them from being fully bent or stretched

CVA cerebrovascular accident – a stroke

Dysarthria slurring of speech, caused by damage to the brain cells or nerve connections that control the speech muscles

Dysphasia difficulty understanding or expressing language

Embolism blockage of a blood vessel by a blood clot, air bubble or other substance that has travelled from somewhere else

Emotional lability rapid mood shifts, usually when people are sad or sentimental; excessive laughing and weeping

GP general practitioner, family doctor

Haemorrhage bleeding

Hemianopia blindness in one-half of the visual field; affects sight in either the left half of each eye or the right half of each eye simultaneously (see p 28)

Hemiparesis incomplete paralysis of one side of the body

Hemiplegia paralysis of one side of the body

Hypertension high blood pressure

Ischaemia a reduced supply of blood to a part of the body

Sclerosis diseased hardening of body tissue (eg hardening of the arteries)

Spasticity occurs when muscles contract and stay contracted. When spasticity occurs in the muscles of a limb, the stronger muscles (the 'anti-gravity' muscles) pull the limb into the characteristic 'spastic' position: the arm is bent at the elbow and the fist clenched up against the shoulder; the leg is straight with a 'dropped' foot

Stenosis abnormal narrowing of a passage in the body

Thrombosis blockage of an artery

Thrombus a solid clot of blood growing on the wall of an artery

TIA Transient Ischaemic Attack, a mini-stroke; its effects last for less than 24 hours – usually less than 30 minutes. Results in a temporary reduction in the blood supply to the brain. Anyone experiencing a TIA should see their doctor because TIAs warn of future possible strokes which could be prevented with proper treatment (see p 8)

Veins tubes that carry the blood from the rest of the body to the heart (see also *Arteries*)

Vessel a tube that carries fluid, especially blood vessels

About Age Concern

Caring for someone who has had a stroke is one of a wide range of publications produced by Age Concern England, the National Council on Ageing. Age Concern cares about all older people and believes later life should be fulfilling and enjoyable. For too many this is impossible. As the leading charitable movement in the UK concerned with ageing and older people, Age Concern finds effective ways to change that situation.

Where possible, we enable older people to solve problems themselves, providing as much or as little support as they need. Our network of 1,400 local groups, supported by 250,000 volunteers, provides community-based services such as lunch clubs, day centres and home visiting.

Nationally, we take a lead role campaigning, parliamentary work, policy analysis, research, specialist information and advice provision, and publishing. Innovative programmes promote healthier lifestyles and provide older people with opportunities to give the experience of a lifetime back to their communities.

Age Concern is dependent on donations, covenants and legacies.

Age Concern England
1268 London Road
London SW16 4ER
Tel: 0181-679 8000

Age Concern Scotland
113 Rose Street
Edinburgh EH2 3DT
Tel: 0131-220 3345

Age Concern Cymru
4th Floor
1 Cathedral Road
Cardiff CF1 9SD
Tel: 01222 371566

Age Concern Northern Ireland
3 Lower Crescent
Belfast BT7 1NR
Tel: 01232 245729

Other books in this series

Choices for the carer of an elderly relative
Marina Lewycka
Being a carer may mean many different things – from living at a distance and keeping a check on things by telephone to taking on a full-time caring role. This book looks at the choices facing someone whose parent or other relative needs care. It helps readers to look at their own circumstances and their own priorities and decide what is the best role for themselves – as well as the person being cared for.
£6.99 0-86242-263-9

Caring for someone who has dementia
Jane Brotchie
Caring for someone with dementia can be physically and emotionally exhausting, and it is often difficult to think about what can be done to make the situation easier. This book shows how to cope better and seek further help as well as containing detailed information on the illness itself and what to expect in the future.
£6.99 0-86242-259-0

Caring for someone who is dying
Penny Mares
Confronting the knowledge that a loved one is going to die soon is always a moment of crisis. And the pain of the news can be compounded by the need to take responsibility for the care and support given in the last months and weeks. This book attempts to help readers cope with their emotions, identify the needs which the situation creates and make the practical arrangements necessary to ensure that the passage through the period is as smooth as possible.
£6.99 0-86242-260-4

The Carer's Handbook: What to do and who to turn to
Marina Lewycka

At some point in their lives millions of people find themselves suddenly responsible for organising the care of an older person with a health crisis. All too often such carers have no idea what services are available or who can be approached for support. This book is designed to act as a first point of reference in just such an emergency, signposting readers on to many more detailed, local sources of advice.

£6.99 0-86242-262-0

Finding and paying for residential and nursing home care
Marina Lewycka

Acknowledging that an older person needs residential care often represents a major crisis for family and friends. Feelings of guilt and betrayal invariably compound the difficulties faced in identifying a suitable care home and sorting out the financial arrangements. This book provides a practical step-by-step guide to the decisions which have to be made and the help which is available.

£6.99 0-86242-261-2

Publications from Age Concern Books

Money matters

Your Rights: A guide to money benefits for older people
Sally West

Written in clear and concise language, *Your Rights* guides readers through the maze of money benefits for older people and explains what you can claim and why. Specific sections are provided on: Retirement Pensions; Housing and Council Tax Benefit; benefits for disabled people; Income Support and the Social Fund; paying for residential care; help with legal and health costs.

For further information please ring 0181-679 8000.

Health and care

The Community Care Handbook: The reformed system explained (2nd edition)
Barbara Meredith

The provision of care in the community is changing as a result of recent legislation. Written by one of the country's foremost experts, this book explains in practical terms the background to the reforms, what they are, how they are working and who they affect.

£13.99 0-86242-171-3

If you would like to order any of these titles, please write to the address below, enclosing a cheque or money order for the appropriate amount made payable to Age Concern England. Credit card orders may be made on 0181-679 8000.

Mail Order Unit
Age Concern England, 1268 London Road, London SW16 4ER

Factsheets from Age Concern

Covering many areas of concern to older people, Age Concern's factsheets are comprehensive and totally up to date. There are over 40 factsheets, with each one providing straightforward information and impartial advice in a simple and easy-to-use format. Topics covered include:

■ finding and paying for residential and nursing home care
■ raising income from your home
■ money benefits
■ legal arrangements for managing financial affairs
■ finding help at home

Single copies are available free on receipt of a 9" × 12" sae.

Age Concern offers a factsheet subscription service which presents all the factsheets in a folder, together with regular updates throughout the year. The first year's subscription currently costs £40; an annual renewal thereafter is £20.

For further information, or to order factsheets, write to:
Information and Policy Division
Age Concern England
1268 London Road
London SW16 4ER

For readers in Scotland wishing further information, or to order factsheets, please write to:

Age Concern Scotland
113 Rose Street
Edinburgh EH2 3DT

Subscribers in Scotland will be automatically sent Scottish editions of factsheets where law and practice differ in Scotland.

Index